Kimberly
Parsons

A Balanced
Life

Align your chakras and find
your best self through yoga
and meditation

Illustrations by Cloudy Thurstag

Hardie Grant

QUADRILLE

PUBLISHING DIRECTOR: Sarah Lavelle
SENIOR COMMISSIONING EDITOR: Céline Hughes
DESIGNER: Alicia House
ILLUSTRATOR: Cloudy Thurstag
HEAD OF PRODUCTION: Stephen Lang
SENIOR PRODUCTION CONTROLLER: Nikolaus Ginelli

Published in 2021 by Quadrille,
an imprint of Hardie Grant Publishing

QUADRILLE
52–54 Southwark Street
London SE1 1UN
quadrille.com

Cataloguing in Publication Data: a catalogue record
for this book is available from the British Library.

Text © Kimberly Parsons 2021
Design and layouts © Quadrille 2021

ISBN 978 1 78713 552 9

Printed in China

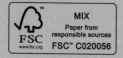

MIX
Paper from
responsible sources
FSC™ C020056
FSC
www.fsc.org

Contents

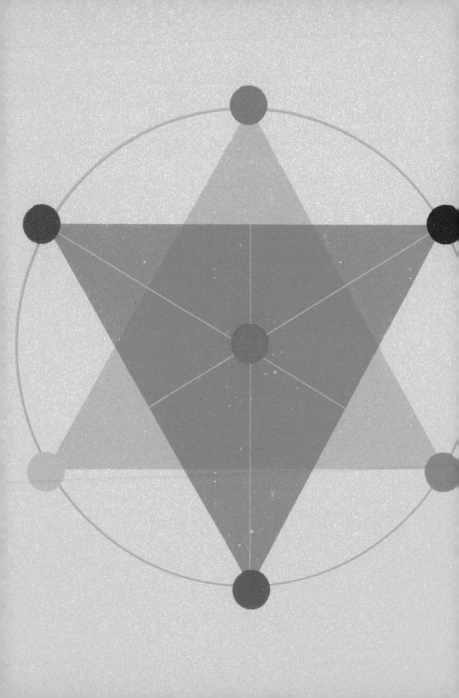

Introduction

Balance – I think we often assume it's something we can achieve all in a day's work. Tick enough things off our to-do list and we will 'get' it, as if it's an object we can hold onto at the end of the day. Some of us treat it like a destination, enjoying the journey towards it by committing to any number of 'wellness' lifestyle techniques and rituals. Others put their path towards balance in the hands of a yoga teacher, personal trainer, doctor, nutritionist or spiritual healer, preferring to offload the responsibility onto someone else.

While we may experience 'balance' for a few fleeting moments, how many of us can honestly say we live a balanced life? Curating a life where balance gets to hang around as a constant participant isn't as easy as we have been led to believe. Too fleeting, too hard, and elusive in nature, balance seems to be something most of us have given up on, leaving it to monks to experience and evangelise.

Far from being a monk myself, like many people I assumed that once I had achieved certain milestones, reached a certain age, meditated for 20 minutes a day, cooked with organic seasonal produce, started a gratitude journal, bought a yoga mat, floated in a salty warm water pod and got rid of those energy vampires,

I too would feel blissfully 'balanced'; wafting through life on a fluffy cloud where none of life's troubles could reach me. Too Zen to notice or just so damn calm and relaxed that I would approach life's disappointments or challenges with Yoda-like skills.

While there have been some Zen-like moments and balance has not been unattainable in my life, for periods of time my ambitious, high-achieving mind-set and frantic lifestyle made it too uninhabitable for balance to move in and get cosy. In fact, at times I could even say that I created a hostile environment for it.

To some degree I thought I knew how to obtain it. Intuition was telling me the answer existed somewhere in the idea of slowing down and embracing a much simpler life, but I decided to ignore it, believing I didn't need it and I would be fine without it, despite feeling stressed, tired and overexposed most of the time.

The moment I decided to turn the boat around and head towards living a more balanced life came in the disguise of maternity leave with my first child. I stopped working every day and started to realise I wasn't going to be able to live my fast-paced lifestyle any more (and if I am completely honest, it was with a large sprinkling of relief). I gave in to the calmer seas of living in a more harmonious way. I even remember writing on my vision board 'I want to live a simple and balanced life as a mother'. #mumgoals

Now, as I sit here and write, I am finding my way through my first year as a new mother. My journey towards granting balance access to my home has been more about doing less than my previous formula allowed, which had always been to do more. As I grappled with the unproductive, selfless and unrelenting days of motherhood, I came to realise the beautiful thing that is balance is actually there for the taking, inside all of us, just waiting to be embraced. Attaining balance happened as a result of needing to live in the present moment with my son and understanding I feel at peace when life is simple and pared back to the seven basic needs I identified and now use as a tool to find balance every day.

My passion for life's natural cycles and rhythms led me to train as a naturopath and learn the art of treating health holistically. For 15 years, my private practice experience has revealed how the increased responsibilities of living a fast-paced life have diminished society's ability to find balance.

These seven basic needs, which I call my 'balance superpowers' and which are discussed in detail in My Balance Superpowers (page 75), are the backbone of how I live my balanced life. They can create the road map to help anyone seeking the same. It doesn't matter if you feel you've just wandered a few feet off the path, or if you're having a few off days but hoping you will feel back to normal soon enough, or if night has fallen on you too many times, leaving you so bewildered that the idea of balance seems like a long-lost relative you don't expect to ever see again. Whatever your circumstances, this book is your practical guide to help you navigate balance, maintain its presence in your life, and shake off the manic lifestyle and headspace that plague our modern lives.

This book's aim is to validate the needs you face physically, mentally and spiritually. It contains something for everyone – theories on the mind, body, spirit (or soul, but I'll refer to it as spirit) and chakra system for the intellectuals, mandala art for the visionaries, meditations for the ethereal, and practical tips for the motivated achievers. Hopefully it will provide solutions, with enlightened thoughts, wisdom and soulful essence you can recreate in your life.

Before we begin…

Whether you're picking this book up for the first time or the hundredth time, I would like to offer you this moment to honour you and the life you are currently living. Give thanks and offer gratitude to where you are today. Take this opportunity to reflect and take stock of where you are, what has passed, and what may have brought you to pick up this book.

Give yourself permission to look back over the last few weeks, months or years and see just how far you've come. If you're not happy with where you are, that's okay. Be kind to yourself – living up to our own expectations can often be our own undoing.

As you read these pages, try to be as honest with yourself as possible – those rose-tinted glasses aren't going to help you get the answers you need here. Remember, this is all about you getting to live your most authentic life in a balanced way.

Seeing life from a different perspective can be the impetus you are looking for to unlock patterns that have been hindering you from living your best life. Approach these pages with a child-like curiosity, which allows you to stay open to all concepts and thoughts for you to mull over. You never know, something may just click into place, blow your mind in the most magical way and give you the renewed energy you've been looking for.

The Balancing Act

You don't need to master everything in the 'Balance is...' list below or aim to achieve all of this all the time. Balance means slightly different things to different people, so not all these 'states' will chime with everyone, but these are my interpretations on the balancing act; you might like to make your own list or adapt mine to suit you.

Balance is...

- Living in the present moment.
- A state of complete calm.
- Feeling grounded, centred and/or at peace.
- Feeling connected to all aspects of myself.
- Feeling liberated from life's mundane chores, free to explore feelings and my passions.
- Living with intention.
- Doing much, much less.
- Aligning my deepest desires with enough energy to support their realisation.
- Constantly evolving and changing.
- Living with my mind, body and spirit in harmony.
- Self-care.

- Having time to do yoga every day.
- Meeting my individual, daily needs while also staying true and connected to myself.
- Meditating for 20 minutes every day.
- Living a simple life where I am able to be present in every moment.
- Multifaceted and often complicated.
- Making sure I am loving me today and staying connected to whatever my mind and body need without the input of anyone else's influence.
- Having all my ducks in a row.
- Being creative, feeling inspired and open to new things.
- Living out my purpose every day.
- Finding the right recipe for the ingredients of life – family, work, love, happiness, stress, anger, sadness, joy, all combined in perfect harmony – when one ingredient is 'spilt', the others are adjusted to maintain the recipe.
- Adjusting to different aspects of my life according to inner and outer influences.
- Feeling content and truly at peace in day-to-day life.
- Time to work, rest and play in equal measure while prioritising self-care.
- Enjoying a simpler life.
- Whatever I decide it to be.
- A skill I chose to learn so I can maintain it daily.
- Deeply personal to me and my individual characteristics.
- Within me.

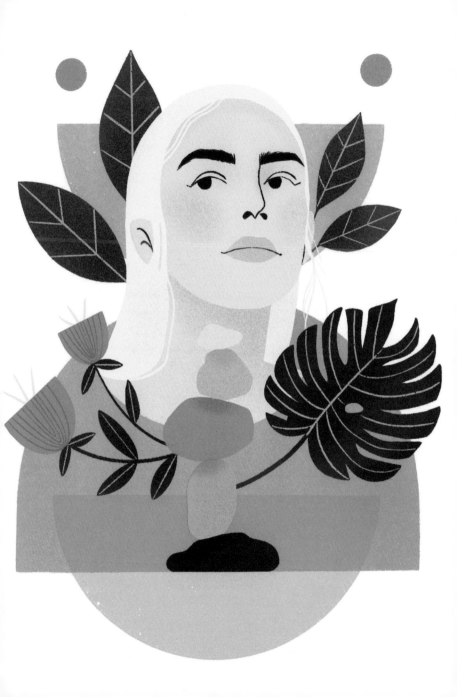

Balance is not...

- Feeling overwhelmed.
- Feeling busy and pulled in many directions.
- Ticking all the things off my to-do list.
- Acting like a slave to my inboxes.
- Idle or static.
- Forcing myself to fit everything into my day so I can feel accomplished.
- Drinking green juice, following a diet and killing myself at the gym every day.
- Productivity.
- Giving up the things that make my heart sing to do the things that don't.
- The same for everyone.
- Achieved by following a pre-determined, run-of-the-mill prescription.
- Ignoring my emotions and focussing on external factors only.
- Reaching a certain status or goal in life.
- Someone else's problem.
- Something I find.
- A destination.
- Simple.

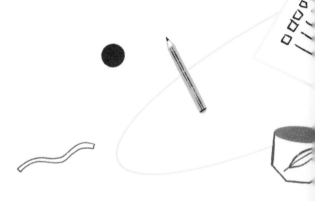

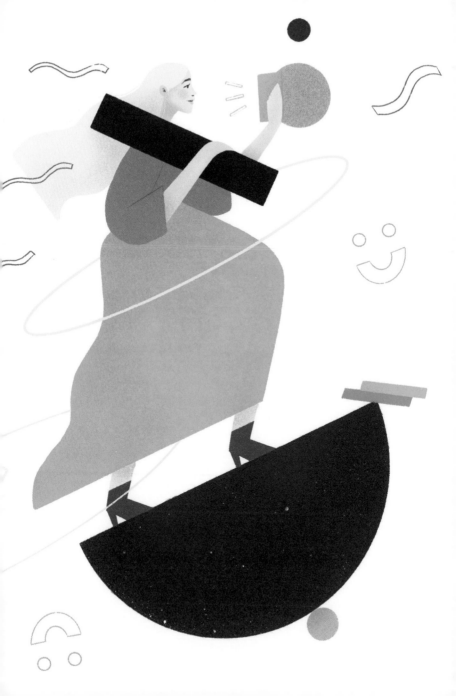

The self-care craze

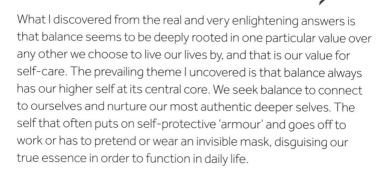

While doing my research for this book I asked
friends, family and my wider community:
'What does balance mean to you?'
'When do you feel the most balanced?'
Or simply, 'What is your definition of balance?'

What I discovered from the real and very enlightening answers is
that balance seems to be deeply rooted in one particular value over
any other we choose to live our lives by, and that is our value for
self-care. The prevailing theme I uncovered is that balance always
has our higher self at its central core. We seek balance to connect
to ourselves and nurture our most authentic deeper selves. The
self that often puts on self-protective 'armour' and goes off to
work or has to pretend or wear an invisible mask, disguising our
true essence in order to function in daily life.

The curse of living in a fast-paced world where we often spend our
worklife fulfilling tasks we don't feel passionate about leads us to
swing strongly towards the extreme of following our passions or
what makes us feel good when we get the time to equalise and
'find balance'. Our pursuit of 'balance' aims to offset the negative
effects of modern living or not living our authentic experience and
seeks to adjust this imbalance with self-care, which, essentially,
seeks to heal our self, the self we neglect and disconnect from.

Although an ancient tradition, the modern-day concept of self-
care somehow only really exploded onto our airwaves right about
the time avocado production tripled in Chile, we heard that Oprah
meditates for 20 minutes every day and noticed that Twitter had

created a self-care bot known as @tinycarebot, who offers gentle reminders to its followers to improve their health and wellbeing by sending them encouraging messages such as 'breathe deeply please' and 'please remember to look up from your screen'.

The baby boomers, Gen-X and now millennials are no strangers to self-care, from the meditation and essential oils of the 60s to the Jane Fonda aerobics tapes of the 1980s and the fat-free-everything 1990s. 'Nothing can bring you peace but yourself,' wrote Ralph Waldo Emerson in 1841, sounding a bit like a modern-day SoulCycle instructor. From these deep roots, the billion-dollar self-care industry has grown.

The influence of technology

Today, like so much around us, the self-care industry is heavily influenced by tech. Focus has shifted away from the actual self – our bodies, minds and spirits – and steered directly towards receiving and analysing data about ourselves. With 'iEverythings' around us at all times, we count our steps, record our REM sleep cycles and measure our breathing patterns. It's not enough to just feel better — now we require tech and our devices to affirm that we are actually doing the self-care legwork. This got me thinking and I found myself asking if this dogged self-care quest is the antidote to our imbalanced lives. Are large sections of society approaching the pursuit of work-life balance with the same obsessive (and oppressive) energy as some of us do our careers?

The American Psychiatric Association reported in 2018 that 39% of US adults felt more anxious than they did in 2017. Yet, despite this rising problem, Americans continue to glamorise being overworked, busy and stressed, wearing these fated titles as a badge of honour. Numerous studies support this research, with the *Journal of Consumer Research* publishing information in 2018 showing that Americans associate busyness and stress with prestige and status (and of course, this mindset isn't limited to the US). This might explain why counting steps and recording exhales are satisfying ways to measure the success of our self-care routine once we leave the office. But in this context, our high anxiety becomes just another thing to 'work on'.

Like most people, I consulted the Google gods when I embarked on my self-care escapade. But endless mindfulness articles, workout regimes and life-coaching ads later, I still hadn't found a super-easy 'how-to' guide that gave me all the answers to how I could simply and effectively find balance or 'do' self-care in a practical way. So like most people, I stumbled along blindly, trying meditation apps, paying attention to my negative thoughts and incorporating nature bathing into my weekly schedule. I kept up my yoga practice and even took a part-time job at Sweaty Betty in the hope that by being around like-minded colleagues I could master this self-care puzzle. But six months into this trial-and-error fling with self-care, I wasn't any closer to cracking the code to finding long-lasting moments of Zen and calm.

I asked myself, 'Is balance completely unachievable?', 'Am I doing self-care all wrong?', 'Do I need to do more of it?', 'If self-care is supposed to help me feel more balanced, why isn't it working?'. I came to realise the answer to my questions lies somewhere in these wise words – we are human 'beings' not human 'doings'! The act of doing more in order to seek balance is a flawed equation, especially if we are spending our days doing things we don't want to be doing and then trying to jam our limited 'down-time' with the things we do love. In my opinion, we have been approaching balance from all the wrong angles and we desperately need a system upgrade, we need Balance 2.0!

Balance 2.0

We are all innately gifted with something called body intelligence – an intuitive sense of what best serves our mental, physical and emotional wellbeing. This innate wisdom gives us specific feedback on how life affects us, from any medication we take to the food we eat, the work we do, the relationships we have. However, most of us disconnect from our body's persistent efforts to communicate, muting it in favour of the breakneck pace of our modern lives. Left unchecked, this can leave us seriously exposed to mental and physical health issues. However, listening to your body is not just about avoiding future illness. It is about wellness, balance and vitality, and about being able to have the life you – and your body – will love now!

As a naturopath, I am fortunate to have the time to really listen to my patients and to hear what is behind their symptoms. I schedule a long session with new patients, to hear about their concerns and complaints in their own words. I learn about their lives in great detail and piece together their manifestation of dis-ease by their body language, body signs and what they say. To me, every patient is like a jigsaw that I need to take apart and put back together.

More often than not I hear my patients tell me they feel pulled in multiple directions by their varied roles and responsibilities. They feel both overwhelmed and exhausted by their many blessings and burdens. These are all symptoms of living in this incredibly prosperous and diverse world, where there are unbelievable opportunities and resources available to us, access to so much information and medical technology, great food and education, yet the western world has never been more depressed, sick, anxious, medicated or obese in the history of humankind.

We live in these beautiful, finely crafted bodies made up of a mind, a body and a spirit – we are capable of phenomenal things – but we forget this body was created for an environment wildly different to the one we now inhabit. We were shaped to live by the sun and the moon with minimal artificial light, to be outside for the majority of the daytime, exposed to natural light and physically active. Now we live in a world where we can do almost none of these things.

Of course I am not suggesting we revert to living as cave men and women, but I do believe we have swung the pendulum too far in the opposite direction. Today, most of us find ourselves indoors all day, sitting at a desk, stressed out, bombarded with text messages, emails and tweets, and told to be productive in order to survive. Then we sit in a car or on a train or bus and head to a home with artificial light, where, exhausted from the stresses of the day, we sit on the sofa and watch television – a life where we are typically not physically active, don't get enough sleep, and feel disconnected and lonely. We live imbalanced lives completely divorced from our existence and expect small occasional acts of self-care to swing the pendulum back the other way, towards health and being at one with our environment.

While self-care can be incredibly calming, nurturing and loving, it does not seek to solve our balance problems. It is simply a symptomatic relief to the even larger problem, which is that for most of us living in a westernised culture, we live vastly imbalanced lives in a fast-paced world and as a result, for some of us, the pressure to maintain a self-care practice and fit it into our already-busy lives seems to be wearing us out even more than the initial problem itself, therefore making a balanced life even less achievable.

It's become clear to me that for many of us, balance can feel like trying to fit a square peg into a round hole. Our lives just don't accommodate its terms and conditions. It's not simple in its nature and often too fleeting and elusive for some of us to want to grapple with. So we give up and soldier on without it. But does it have to be this way? If you had a simple-to-use framework you could follow, that promised to lead you easily in the right direction towards living a balanced life, would you use it?

The way forward

So, let's take balance and turn it on its head! Let's redesign it with real integrity, heart and soul. Work out what's been missing and why we haven't yet been able to utilise the concept of balance in our day-to-day lives in a meaningful way. Forget focusing on things we can 'do', 'acquire' or 'control' – these are external factors that simply distract from the real issue. Instead, we should be asking ourselves, 'How do I want to feel?'. By answering that question, we enable our true desires to speak for us, allowing us the freedom to explore what sets our soul on fire and how we can truly live the balanced life we crave.

Remember, our goal is to allow balance to move in, get cosy and become a guest whom you love having around all the time because they make you feel comforted, relaxed and genuinely excited. Not the annoying one-night guests who don't clean up after themselves, want a home-cooked meal waiting for them, drink your expensive wine, and then leave you feeling totally exhausted! Excuse the bad analogy, but I hope you get my point – that's not the kind of balance I want in my life and certainly not what I want for you either! Rather, I'd much prefer you feel calm, grounded, purposeful, motivated and centred. I want you to feel you have a handle on the various elements in your life without your heart or mind being pulled too hard in any direction.

I truly believe that living a balanced life is not a prescription you can Google; it's a skill set you must learn. Simply looking around to see what the latest trends are and following someone else's choices will not make you happy, healthy or balanced. The key to health, happiness and living a balanced life is to find out how you and your body function and what you and your body crave. To find out what you truly desire and need in order for you to feel centred and calm regardless of what someone else's pursuits may entail. Honour your individuality and #justdoyou.

It is my mission to help you honour your individuality and 'do you' by offering you the framework to set you on the road towards living your most authentic, balanced life. You will learn all the navigation skills, so you will always be able to find your way and know where you are. Life can then take on a simplicity that avoids confusion, burden and stress, and most importantly doesn't make you want to give up. #whenyouknowbetteryoudobetter – thanks Oprah!

The Chakra Rainbow

For many of us, our journey towards living a balanced life doesn't look anything like the #balancedlife Instagram posts we see of candlelit bubble baths or yoga poses to the backdrop of dazzling sunsets. While some of us may have been lucky enough to live balanced lives during our childhood and teenage years, all too often we somehow lose it into adulthood. By 'it' I mean we lose that sweet simplicity of being allowed to just... be – free to do what we like and live with minimal responsibilities. Of course we learn coping strategies to survive manically busy lifestyles, relentless workloads and the burdens of modern life, but we sure as hell aren't teleporting ourselves to any island paradise where we get to live happy, healthy and balanced lives.

My turning point

With hindsight, I can now see what was missing in times I have lived an imbalanced life. For most of my life, I have certainly had purpose, but I was missing a strong connection to myself, I wasn't 'in tune' with my daily needs for calm, balance and health. I didn't have that little radar going off each time I hit a damaging new limit, telling me to slow down or change things up. Instead, the constant ON-switch meant that when something happened in my day-to-day life that shook me, I didn't know how to circumnavigate or process it without it leaving some sort of lasting impact.

Over time, these small but significant little impacts took their toll and I crumbled. I just gave it all up! Just like that. I sold my business, moved to the countryside where I could see blue skies and green surroundings and just stopped dead in my tracks for a while. I did it relatively quietly (my ego didn't want the world knowing I had 'given-up/dropped-the-ball/caved' – all of those terms felt like failure). I stopped answering my phone and let my inbox fill up while I hibernated and contemplated my next move! I took an extended three-month trip to spend time with friends and family in Australia and basically got my sh*t sorted.

In the process of 'getting my sh*t sorted' I did a lot of soul searching. I asked myself questions like 'How do I want to feel?' instead of 'What do I want to achieve?'. I decided I needed a new approach to how I lived my daily life. On re-entry into my life in England, I was more determined than ever to live a more balanced and simplified life. By some miracle I was invited to a yoga retreat run by the formidable force that is Lizaan Joubert. I call her my 'truth compass' because she always sends me the most amazing #truthbombs – shooting them straight from the hip with piercing accuracy and intense heart-felt intuition. It was her chakra mapping workshops that led to my lightbulb moment.

My dedication to the chakras had been developing over the years, I had been writing recipes using them, learning about the persona and application of each individual chakra, but I hadn't quite cracked how the chakras interacted and worked together as a unified system until Lizaan offered her wisdom and literally spoke a language I fully and passionately understood and could apply to my life. It was simple – the chakras were the perfect navigating system I had been seeking to help me live a more balanced life. I immediately realised if all the colours aren't present and in harmony, there simply is no rainbow. Each chakra is integral and part of a profound and larger structure that holds mind, body and spirit in perfect harmony – a beautiful sacred framework that offered a lens through which I could look at life and the world around me. It was a revelation and I started calling it my 'Chakra Rainbow'.

What is the Chakra Rainbow?

The Chakra Rainbow consists of seven basic human needs, which I call my 'balance superpowers'. The chakra system is an organisational centre for the reception, assimilation and transmission of the energy flowing through your mind, body and spirit. These seven chakras represent your energetic architecture and are part of the subtle body, which comprises your psychological, emotional and spiritual states of being.

I am all too aware our western culture, too pragmatic and scientific to accept things on faith, has lost touch with the world of spirit and the sense of unity it can bring. Ancient systems, couched in language and tradition so different from our own, are often too alienating for the western mind. But in order for you to believe or put any faith in this Chakra Rainbow, you first have to accept the idea that your body is not only made up of what you can physically see but also what you can feel. Accept you are a living human being who lives within a dynamic and integrated trilogy of mind, body and spirit. Mind is where your thoughts, emotions and behaviour are governed; body is your biological, physical makeup; and spirit is the vital principle or animating force within all living things, where energy binds the soul to the body.

As Marion Woodman, a Canadian psychologist and author, named the 100th most spiritually influential living person by *Mind Body Spirit* magazine in 2012, put it: 'Matter without spirit is a corpse. Spirit without matter is a ghost.' Demonstrating that in order to be fully alive, to feel, to have emotions and desires, we require both physical matter of the mind and body and a spirit.

While at university, where I studied to be a naturopath, I was surrounded by people who not only accepted but were also establishing careers based on the very existence of the mind, body and spirit theory. We accepted it just as we accepted the concept of gravity. It just was! A trilogy that needed to be honoured and recognised in all human beings in order to practise true holistic medicine and help patients find equilibrium through all three elements. When I went home, I would witness my mother's work as a clairvoyant, medium and spiritual healer. She would clear 'bad energy' and help her clients connect to spirit energy around them in order to heal emotional wounds and find peace. You see, I have never not known a world where the mind, body and spirit didn't exist. To me, they just are – just as I have two arms, I also have my mind, my body and my spirit.

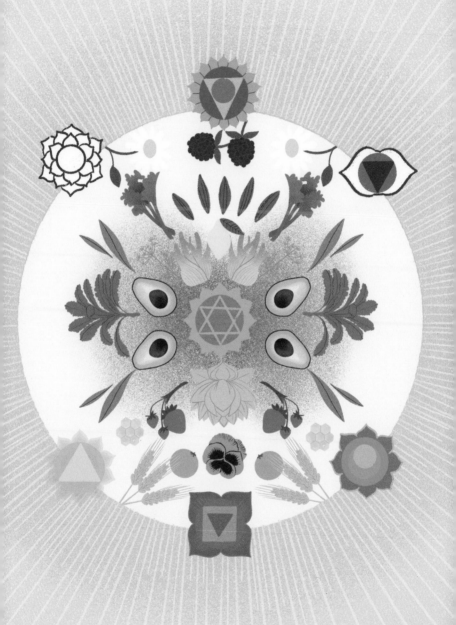

Ten things you need to know about chakras

1. The Sanskrit word *chakra* translates literally to 'sacred wheel' or 'disk'. The life-force energy (also known as *chi* or *prana*) that moves inside you is constantly spinning and rotating. This clockwise spinning energy has seven main wheels (chakras) in your body, starting at the base of your spine, moving up to the top of your head. These swirling wheels of energy correspond to dense areas of nerve activity (nerve ganglia) and major organs within the body – a network of 72,000 channels (called *nadi* in Sanskrit, which translates as 'tubes' or 'pipes') that conduct an energetic life force throughout our body. These energy channels form a nerve network and meet in seven major confluences, known as the chakras.

2. The lower three chakras (root, sacral and solar plexus) all pertain to the physical body, while the heart chakra sits in the middle with limbs in both the physical and spiritual bodies. The top three chakras (throat, third eye and crown) all pertain to psychological and spiritual aspects of us.

3. More than four thousand years ago, the ancient yogis of India described a second, subtler nervous system that exists alongside our physical nervous system. The seven chakras represent that energetic anatomy and are part of the subtle body, which comprises our physical, energetic, emotional, mental and spiritual states of being. They are linked to certain emotions, qualities, modes of thinking and feeling, behaviours, ego and different states of consciousness, including the most spiritual ones. This means each chakra corresponds to aspects of our human experience, such as our ability for love, compassion and forgiveness, our willpower, ambition and personal identity, perception of ourselves and the world around us, intuition and self-expression through speech and creativity, plus so much more.

4. Chakras do not function independently of each other or of the physical mind or body, but rather as the gears in the larger human experience – the mind, body and spirit. They work together as a unified system and should be considered a family unit of seven members who all work together.

5. Since chakras exist in the space between spirit and matter, at the energetic level of human existence, they can easily become clogged or dense due to emotional, mental, energetic and spiritual factors. The optimal activity of the chakras can be hindered by diet, stress, electromagnetic disturbances, inner issues triggered by certain circumstances and also the condition of our loved ones' chakras.

6. Through involvement with the outside world, patterns within the chakras tend to perpetuate themselves; hence the idea of karma – patterns formed through action, or the laws of cause and effect. Thus it is common to become trapped in any one of these patterns. This is called being 'stuck' in a chakra. We are caught in a cycle that keeps us at a particular level. This could be a relationship, job, habit, but most often, simply a way of thinking. Being stuck can be a function of either overemphasis or underdevelopment of a chakra. The object of our work is to clean the chakra of the old, non-beneficial patterns so that their self-perpetuating actions have a positive influence and our life energy can continue to expand to higher planes.

7. Each chakra has the ability to give us an unbelievable amount of energy and power if in alignment and we tune into it. Remember, chakra energy centres are often thought of as vortexes or wheels of energy, spinning just as the stars and planets rotate. But, if one of your chakras spins too quickly (excessive/ overemphasis), is left too 'open', is blocked, or moves slowly (deficient/underdeveloped), you can feel out of balance, and lethargy and powerlessness can develop. Think of the chakras like the wheels and cogs of a car engine. The car has an optimal speed for conserving energy and avoiding too much wear and tear. If we drive too fast, it burns through the fuel, eventually running out of energy to keep it going while putting extra stress on its functioning parts. If we drive the car at a pace slower than its preferred optimum pace, then the car will take longer to reach its destination and never reach a temperature that warms the engine or tyres enough to function properly. This metaphor demonstrates that chakras like to spin at their individual optimal rate, so if a chakra gets 'stuck' in either an open or closed state, its rotation slows down and it sends a far smaller amount of energetic nourishment to the physical systems that surround it. This chakra then needs to be rebalanced and healed by uncovering and removing whatever is blocking it. If the chakra is not unblocked, this energy becomes stagnant and physical symptoms can manifest in the body. Negative emotions and physiological states can develop, leading to you experiencing the negative aspects of that particular chakra.

8. In a healthy, balanced person, the seven chakras provide the right balance of energy to every part of your body, mind and spirit, offering positive attributes cohesive to feeling balanced, energised and whole. Healing, balancing and opening the chakra system mark major life stages and phases in our emotional maturation, the crystallisation of our wisdom of life, as well as our spiritual progress. It is through the chakra system that we can transform and become an awakened spirit.

9. Chakras correspond to a certain colour, element or symbol, as well as many more touch points such as body parts, endocrine organs, gemstones, seasons and planets. The link between the chakras and their specific colours is much more than mere symbolism. When we shine pure white light through a crystal or if we look at a rainbow, the white light divides into its primary colours. Each colour corresponds to a certain wavelength of light, a frequency of energy. In view of this, we could say that each colour seems to have a certain physical wavelength that affects our body and psyche in a unique way. Accordingly, the colours appear in the chakra system in an ascending order of their wavelength – starting with the lowest frequency in the first chakra up to the highest frequency in the crown.

10. The seven chakras are a clear outline of all levels of human existence and development – beginning with the most earthly levels of instinct, impulse and our basic relationship with life on Earth (root chakra), and culminating in our most refined layers of higher mental faculties and connection with the infinite source of life (crown chakra). In this, they capture our journey of transcendence along which we overcome what is known as 'the challenge', or limitations and inhibitions of each chakra. Eventually, if we are able to 'master' the challenge, we unlock 'the right' of that chakra, enabling spiritual states of being, which demonstrate fearlessness, unconditional love, and a vast and expanded sense of self.

The purpose of the Chakra Rainbow

You can use this as a checklist to refer back to, if you are finding the process difficult at times or have lost your way and need to remind yourself of its benefits and potential.

1. Ultimately, to remind you that you are a beautiful soul with individual needs and characteristics that set you apart from anyone else.

2. To offer a solution to unwanted emotions and daily struggles.

3. To show you a way to listen to your mind, body and soul. Find out what they need and work out what core desires you feel you need for balance, health and empowerment.

4. Perhaps, most importantly, to understand what your mind, body and soul don't like and what hinders their potential and wellness.

5. To help accentuate your positive aspects while still honouring and not invalidating the negative aspects of you that you would like to change, acknowledging that you are an imperfect being who is constantly balancing your own equilibrium.

6. To help you piece together the parts of yourself that make up a much larger picture and create the whole you – an ever-evolving individual with a vital force, spirit and core feelings which are individual to you and make you who you are.

7. To give you the tools to be your own captain of the ship with stellar navigation tools so you never feel lost at sea ever again.

All the Colours
of the Rainbow

Once you start to understand the personality
of each chakra, you will be able to see yourself
reflected in them and build a picture of your own
psyche through them. Understanding which
chakras dominate and drive your persona, while
also defining which chakras may need some
attention and rebalancing, is an essential step.

It's important to remember that the energy
contained in the subtle body – our chakras –
is formed by learnt habits over many years.
Therefore, some chakras may take years to
rebalance as you retrain your mind and body to act
and think differently. Equally, some chakras can
be rebalanced in just a few moments by bringing
attention to them and changing the energy.

Root Chakra

The Root of Security
Grounding • Safety • Community

Overview

Persona: Home sweet home

Sanskrit name: *Muladhara*

Meaning: Root support

Colour: Red

Season: Late summer

Sense: Smell

Element: Earth

Energy: Masculine

Psychological function: Survival

Resulting in: Grounding

Identity: Physical identity

Qualities: Instinctual trust, patience, diligence, responsibility, practicality, orderliness, efficiency, accuracy

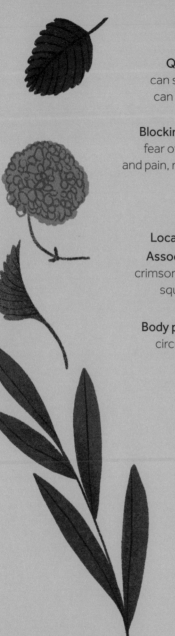

Quest: A safe ground on which one can solidly stand, a home to which one can belong – on the planet, with one's family and within one's body

Blocking fears: A general mistrust of life, fear of change, physical danger, disease and pain, natural disasters, physical violence and abuse, poverty, aloneness

Rights: To have

Challenge: Fear

Location: Base of the spine, perineum

Associated symbol: A four-petal, deep crimson lotus flower, at its core is a yellow square, symbol of the Earth element

Planets: Saturn and Earth

Body parts: Bone and muscle structure, circulatory system and large intestine

The balanced root chakra

A person whose root chakra is balanced feels healthy and at home in their body, in this world, and has developed an inner sense of security and stability, independent of ever-changing circumstances. They allow themselves to flow with life's changes because they have found stability inside themselves and trust life at a much deeper level. Thus, such a person builds on life's experiences happily and joyfully, and will establish foundations and solid structures like purchasing a residential home, long-term relationship/s, steady work, a steady income, while remaining worry-free. Such a person would remain responsible, aware of consequences and of future calculations, while being flexible enough to manage and even welcome change. The most existential and instinctual fears, worries and anxieties would not overshadow their ability to relax and enjoy life.

A balanced root chakra also provides a deep sense of belonging and community. The person has a strong tribal mentality, recognising they feel safe and secure when they have a place they can define as 'home' – be it a family, a person, a country, house or faith – this sense of 'home' offers support, trust and the very foundations of this person's life. It is their metaphorical 'anchor' they can keep coming back to in life when change occurs and they need to recentre and find stability again.

The imbalanced root chakra

An imbalanced root chakra leads to a general feeling or impression that life is unsafe, unreliable and untrustworthy. This leads to the attempt to generate a sense of security and stability on a material and social level by controlling life, or to the exact opposite – the inability to trust or commit to anything at all.

The direct reflection of this state is the constant stream of thoughts and emotions, which attempts to control and manipulate the uncontrollable – the mind of a constant 'worrier' – caused by fear: that things might change in an undesired way and that they will face unexpected or unwanted change. This results in the person intensely invested in trying to maintain the status quo or properly preparing for a change that might never happen.

Such a blocked state expresses itself when this person may attempt to meditate: they may try to ease the mind and body into being present in the moment, but they are so conditioned to their worries, fears and need to control the future that relaxation is quite impossible. Denial, clinginess and phobias are also characteristics of an imbalanced root chakra.

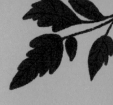

Transcending the root chakra

In this chakra, it's all about feeling safe and trusting life: how much change can we endure, and can we trust life despite its constant changing nature? Can we let life flow and rely on it enough so that we build our structures, maintain our sense of safety *while* accepting its changing nature?

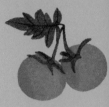

For example, if we are made redundant from our job – creating worry for basic needs such as paying the mortgage or rent, putting food on the table and paying bills – will we be able to trust that someone or a company won't do the same again and push away the impression that you can't ever expect to have job security enough that you are willing to put yourself forward for another job. This example is valid also for our relationships: can we ever trust enough to build a long-term relationship after a previous unexpected break-up? And can we trust our body once again after an unexpected illness or injury?

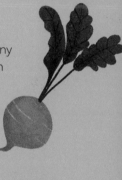

Building a sense of trust, despite the constant changing nature of life, is the main psychological theme of the root chakra: relaxing in our own bodies, in our own home, in our own routine, while maintaining this delicate thread of knowing that no routine, no body, no home can last forever.

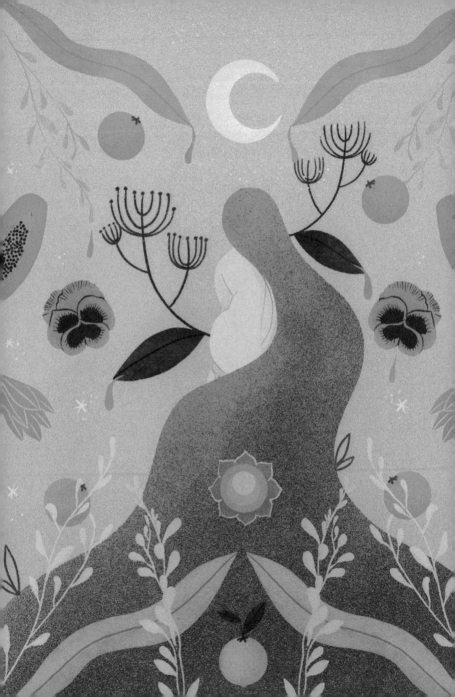

Sacral Chakra
The Seed of Creation
Creativity • Vitality • Sexuality

Overview

Persona: With flow we go

Sanskrit name: *Svadhisthana*

Meaning: Dwelling place of the self

Colour: Orange

Season: Winter

Sense: Taste

Element: Water

Energy: Feminine

Psychological function: Desire

Resulting in: Sexuality

Identity: Emotional identity

Qualities: Vitality, pleasure, joy, flexibility, playfulness, enthusiasm, passion, curiosity, vitality

Quest: A joy of life that lasts

Blocking fears: Moral shame, the pain of disappointment, inner desires

Rights: To feel, to want

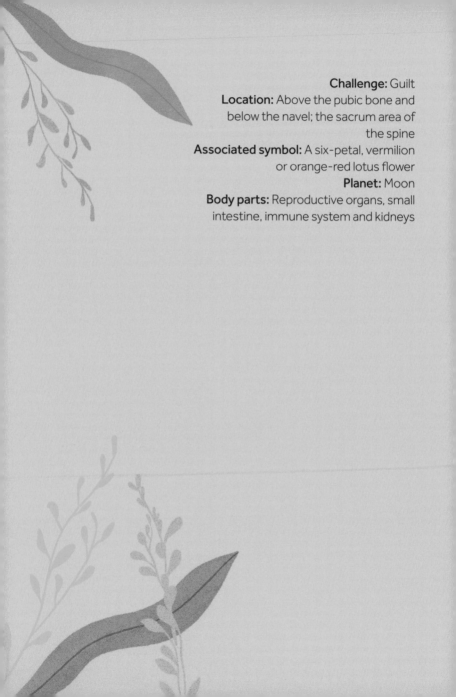

Challenge: Guilt
Location: Above the pubic bone and below the navel; the sacrum area of the spine
Associated symbol: A six-petal, vermilion or orange-red lotus flower
Planet: Moon
Body parts: Reproductive organs, small intestine, immune system and kidneys

The balanced sacral chakra

A balanced sacral chakra leads to a peaceful, yet passionate love for being alive. It provides a constant sense of vibrating joy, passion, excitement and liveliness that is not dependent on certain experiences that come and go.

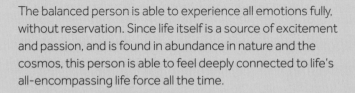

The balanced person is able to experience all emotions fully, without reservation. Since life itself is a source of excitement and passion, and is found in abundance in nature and the cosmos, this person is able to feel deeply connected to life's all-encompassing life force all the time.

A person whose sacral chakra is open has a deep conscious acceptance for their natural needs and desires and does not suppress them with guilt or shame, yet they are not dominated by unconscious obsessions and desires.

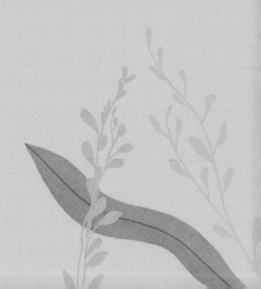

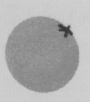

The imbalanced sacral chakra

An imbalanced or blocked sacral chakra is expressed by an intense lack of a person's interest in life – loss of joy, passion, enthusiasm and the ability to feel anything deeply. Their zest for life has all but vanished and they have become numb to all pleasure and emotion.

As such, life becomes boring and only defined by a set of duties and pressures. Everything is seen as a chore, approached with a mechanical and artificial attitude. Delicious food might be consumed, but without any pleasure; sexual indulgence might be experienced in abundance, but without true joy.

Transcending the sacral chakra

The second chakra connects us to the joy and wonder of life. Thus the psychological themes of the sacral chakra are determined by our relationship to life's excitements – peak experiences, intense feelings, adventures, creative ventures, surprises, new revelations and new opportunities – expressed through enjoyment, passion and desire without the scale tipping towards excessive or compulsive indulgence, leading to obsession or addiction. The psychological learning within our second chakra is the cultivation of positive passion, which leads us to find enjoyment, beauty and excitement in the healthy range of life's experiences – and finally in existence itself.

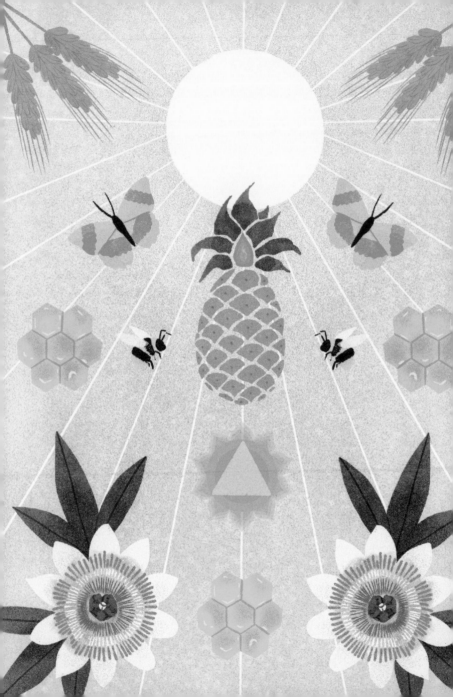

Solar Plexus
Our Warrior Energy
Willpower • Joy • Ambition

Overview

Persona: Your warrior

Sanskrit name: *Manipura*

Meaning: Lustrous gem

Colour: Yellow

Season: Summer

Sense: Sight

Element: Fire

Energy: Masculine

Psychological function: Will

Resulting in: Power

Identity: Ego identity

Qualities: Will, power, identity, ambition, excellence, determination, courage, independence, confidence, resilience, self-dignity

Quest: Finding out what one really wants and what one's sources of strength are

Blocking fears: Fear of failure, social resistance, pressure, rejection, authorities, the danger of possessing 'too much power'

Rights: To act

Challenge: Shame

Location: Around the navel in the area of the solar plexus and up to the breastbone

Associated symbol: A ten-petal, bright yellow lotus flower

Planets: Sun and Mars

Body parts: Adrenal glands, stomach, pancreas, liver and skin

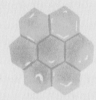

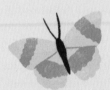

The balanced solar plexus

A balanced solar plexus is characterised by the ability to integrate ambition, desire and other forces that drive our willpower into a congruent, purposeful self, with resolute direction, able to make conscious decisions and define clear, achievable goals. This allows you to have a healthy confidence as a person, know your strengths and weaknesses, and have a realistic understanding of your capabilities and power.

A person with a balanced solar plexus likes to feel challenged and can easily set a goal and follow it through with determination. Even when faced with external pressures, obstacles and difficulties, they are not easily swayed and are able to stay focussed until the task is accomplished, as they do not fear failure but accept it as an inevitable part of the game of life. A person with a healthy solar plexus is unlikely to get distracted by emotions and is stable, reliable, calm, concentrated and considerate, even in stressful situations.

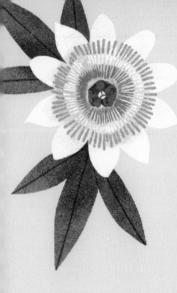

The imbalanced solar plexus

An imbalanced third chakra is characterised by a feeling of powerlessness, often leading to procrastination and the person giving up on their pursuits, no matter how menial.

People who have not opened their third chakra often lack self-discipline, integrity and the willpower to set goals, while others with excessive solar plexus energy might vehemently strive for their goals with dogmatic determination and persistence, leading to burnout and negative traits such as manipulation, intimidation and cheating.

Transcending the solar plexus

The solar plexus acts as the mediator between our instincts, urges, impulses, wishes and outer pressures, expectations and demands. It is strongly related to the Freudian concept of the ego, where mastering our own power and knowing how to act and react to the world around us become the central missions of this chakra.

When people lack the ability to master their power they may experience low self-esteem, low self-respect and the inability to define their own identity. They struggle to answer the question 'What do I want?' and therefore feel too weak to act, become susceptible to others' wills and expectations and are often unable to make their own decisions. They feel frustrated that they don't seem to be able to shape and influence their fate, allowing people and events to influence their path in life. However, if there is an excess of will and power, this can easily turn into an aggressive approach to move life in an obstinate manner.

In order to transcend the solar plexus, the person must accept and adopt a healthy limit to their productivity and ambition, knowing when to stop 'pushing' and instead to allow the natural flow of things.

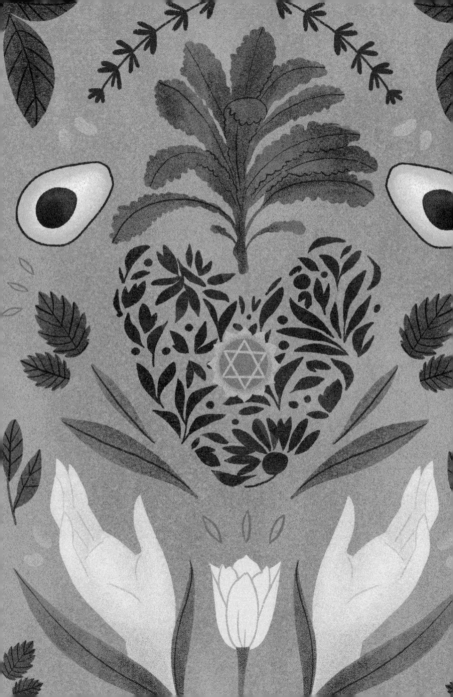

Heart Chakra
The Embodiment of Love
Compassion • Love • Gratitude

Overview

Persona: Love conquers all

Sanskrit name: *Anahata*

Meaning: Unstruck

Colour: Green

Season: Spring

Sense: Touch

Element: Air

Energy: Feminine

Psychological function: Love

Resulting in: Peace

Identity: Social identity

Qualities: Love, generosity, dedication, empathy, compassion, trust, acceptance, forgiveness

Quest: The search for true love – at first outside oneself and then gradually deep within oneself

Blocking fears: Abandonment, rejection, losing oneself in another

Rights: To love

Challenge: Grief

Location: At the centre of the chest

Associated symbol: A twelve-petal lotus flower containing two interlaced triangles and with green petals

Planet: Venus

Body parts: Lungs, heart, thymus glands and breasts

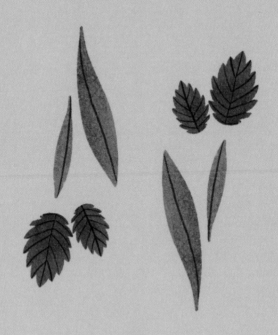

The balanced heart chakra

A balanced heart chakra fills a person with the characteristics of compassion and acceptance – acceptance of one's own weaknesses and limitations, one's own natural constitution and human capacities. This leads to the ability to accept others for their perfect imperfections, without the need to fall into judgement or comparison.

An open-heart chakra heart remains receptive despite betrayal and disappointment. Such a heart does not hold a grudge; it easily forgives and keeps on believing in people's potential and their chance to grow and change.

Such a state of an unconditionally open heart is far from vulnerable, as one might expect. Instead, it is both sensitive and indestructible (hence the name *Anahata*, Sanskrit for unharmed or unbeaten): with an open heart, one would experience complete composure, enabling feeling without fragility.

The imbalanced heart chakra

An imbalanced heart chakra is characterised by emotional dependency. The person does not feel complete within themself and is therefore in a constant struggle with comparison – experienced through love or hate, grudge and bitterness, or attachment and admiration.

This state of dependency causes one to look for the 'perfect' in others, and whenever someone seems to momentarily be able to play this role, this imbalanced heart chakra releases countless projections, expectations, demands and imperfections to be seen and felt within themselves. Fear of abandonment always accompanies such a dependent heart. Sometimes this dependency is masked by overtly independent behaviour, signifying that they 'do not need anybody'. This is only to protect themselves from the same fear of abandonment and is used to anticipate the inevitable disappointment and betrayal from those around them.

Giving is always done in a transactional manner – meaning they give in order to receive – and subtle negotiation is constantly present in the love they do give, so their love is always conditional.

Transcending the heart chakra

The psychological theme of the fourth chakra concerns the right balance between the need to be loved, accepted and have our needs recognised by others, while being able to give love unconditionally.

A mature heart is capable of giving love without feeling 'But what about me?'. It doesn't feel drained by the act of giving, but filled up.

Therefore, psychologically speaking, the heart chakra is all about emotional maturity: growing towards the capacity to fully love and give, including loving oneself without the need for external gratification.

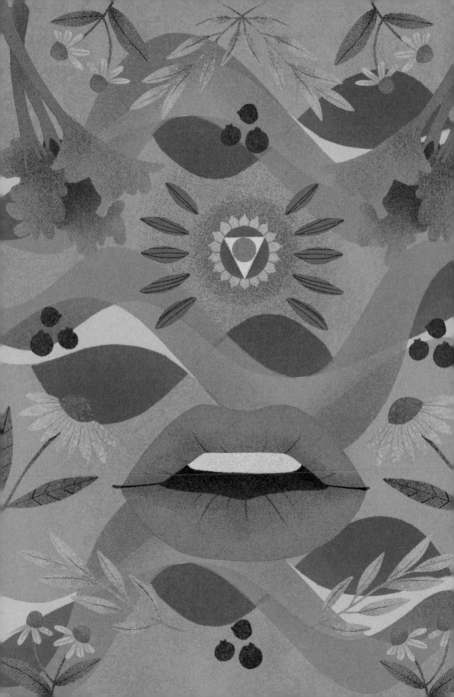

Throat Chakra
The Clear Waters of Communication
Self-expression • Truth • Authenticity

Overview

Persona: The truth will set you free

Sanskrit name: *Vissudha*

Meaning: Purification

Colour: Bright blue

Season: No associated season

Sense: Hearing

Element: Sound, ether

Energy: Masculine

Psychological function: Communication

Resulting in: Creativity

Identity: Creative identity

Qualities: Authenticity, purity, truthfulness, clarity, influence, idealism, receptivity, peace

Quest: The search for truth and the ideal and most authentic expression and fulfilment of one's innermost being

Blocking fears: Fear of rejection, criticism, indifference and injustice

Rights: To speak and be heard

Challenge: Lies

Location: Area around the throat

Associated symbol: A sixteen-petal lotus flower with a white centre depicting a white circle to represent the element ether; blue petals

Planet: Mercury

Body parts: Throat, thyroid and parathyroid glands, immune and lymphatic systems; ears, jaw, mouth, tongue, larynx, shoulders and neck

The balanced throat chakra

When the throat chakra is balanced, it becomes a pure channel for our inner truth. However, this does not mean that a person with a balanced throat chakra carelessly says whatever crosses their mind and heart. On the contrary, this means they know exactly what they want to convey from their inner world, when and how. They have perfectly mastered the process of self-expression and translation. Words, artistic expression or outer gestures are masterfully selected to interact in the right moment, with the right person, in the right way. There is not too much overflow of expression, or too little. It is suited for the needs of their environment and everyone around them.

When the throat chakra is balanced, it becomes less and less self-centred. The inner world is not expressed for its own sake but rather in service. This causes the development of a great sensitivity in interaction: knowing when to be honest, polite and diplomatic; when to influence and direct another, and when quiet and a listening ear are all that is needed.

Becoming a channel, the balanced throat chakra finally brings a person closer to becoming the free-flowing portal where the energy of the soul can freely come out and be expressed.

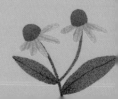

The imbalanced throat chakra

The imbalanced state of the fifth chakra is that of suffocation. A blockage here is caused mainly by an inability to speak, think and live in alignment with our personal highest truth. The shy, quiet observer may be unable to express their inner authentic world, resulting in their truth never being known to their outer environment. The chatterbox may perpetuate their imbalanced throat chakra by constantly speaking but without clarity of thought or authenticity, scared of silence because in these moments they must accept their inner truths, which they may be trying to desperately hide from view with small talk.

People with an imbalanced fifth chakra may fear expressing their truth and it having little or no impact on their desired audience, or perhaps the message becoming confused, leading to an even deeper frustration of being unheard and unrecognised. Perhaps there has been an attempt to express needs, wishes, dreams and understandings authentically, and the result was ridicule and embarrassment; perhaps our unique individuality was severely criticised or we faced a seeming injustice, in which we could not properly defend our truth. All these negative imprints upon the throat chakra leave the impression that our truth is not enough and we are not worthy of acknowledgement.

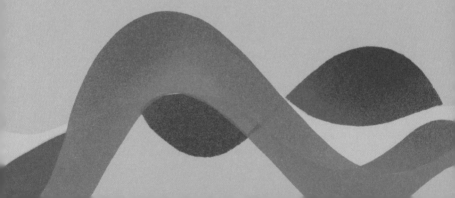

Transcending the throat chakra

The main psychological theme of the throat chakra is how much we can fearlessly and clearly express our inner world of deeper feelings and truths to the world. Our lower chakras (from the root chakra all the way up to the heart chakra) accumulate many feelings, experiences, emotions and wills, and along with our sixth chakra (the third eye) which develops beliefs, convictions and understandings; eventually all this needs to be expressed and voiced. Sometimes, this gateway or bridge seems to be blocked or broken; if the person is unable to express themselves, this can result in a deep separation between the inner and the outer worlds – meaning the person knows themselves with utter conviction but is unable to share themselves with the people around them.

To transcend this chakra we are compelled to overcome our fears and inhibitions, and to speak clearly, honestly and authentically. This can be as simple as knowing how to express our needs and wills, our sorrow, but also our happiness and expressions of love. It can also be the more demanding type of expression and manifestation. Can we give the right form to our dreams and visions, ideals and knowledge? Here again we are challenged to take all that we have gathered and learned and to give it a form that others can understand and be influenced by. This can take place through the different arts or different forms of teaching, lecturing and even manifesting projects that lead to public influence. In summary, if our truth is not expressed, we might remain in a sense of suffocation and frustration in our throat chakra.

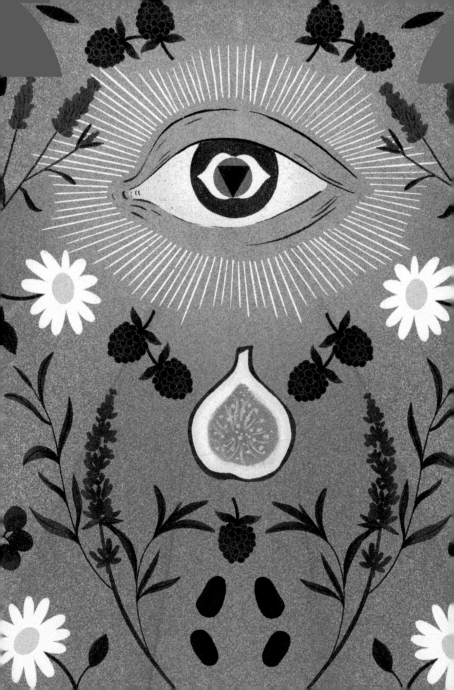

Third-eye Chakra
The All-seeing Intuition
Perception • Wisdom • Imagination

Overview

Persona: The power of the mind

Sanskrit name: *Ajna*

Meaning: Command centre

Colour: Indigo

Season: No associated season

Sense: Mind

Element: Light

Energy: Feminine

Psychological function: Intuition

Resulting in: Imagination

Identity: Archetypal identity

Qualities: Realistic, watchful, attentive, perceptive, curious, silent, intuitive

Quest: The quest for the most reliable source of knowledge and wisdom, as one's source of solid truth

Blocking fears: Disorientation, confusion, not knowing what is true

Rights: To see

Challenge: Illusion

Location: Forehead, between the eyebrows

Associated symbol: Two-petal lotus, one represents the moon and the other, the sun. Within the lotus, a round circle symbolises the void. Within the circle, an inverted triangle representing Shakti, and above it a Shivalingam; indigo petals

Planets: Jupiter and Neptune

Body parts: Brain, eyes, base of skull, brow and pituitary gland

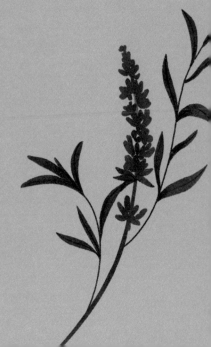

The balanced third-eye chakra

The balanced third-eye establishes our intuition, which can be described as witnessing or a crystal-clear light of awareness that is non-conceptual and unbiased. Precisely because of this clarity, a person whose third-eye is open and balanced has a natural capacity to discriminate through observation – to look at themselves and rely on the highest forms of knowledge to tell reality from illusion.

On the other hand, despite all knowledge, understanding and discrimination, the open third-eye is also deeply non-conceptual. Its centre is in a state of spacious and unlimited listening. It is observant and lucid rather than automatic and reactive – a state which allows a person to be a receptor of 'higher', untainted inner guidance, as well as deep intuition and even super-sensory perception.

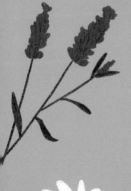

The imbalanced third-eye chakra

The imbalanced sixth chakra can appear as too conceptual, analytical and rigid, or too mentally feeble and fluid. Born out of the fear of not being sure of oneself, this can make one's third eye seem arrogant, but also fearfully unstable and constantly in search of clarity.

To overcome this blocked state and to reach an authentic inner conviction, the person needs to rely on higher forms of knowledge, enter silence and develop deeper capacities of quiet inner observation. At the same time, they also need to fearlessly face confusion and to realise that it is really an opportunity for achieving a deeper, more stable and grounded type of clarity.

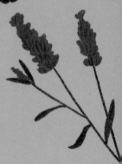

Transcending the third-eye chakra

The psychological themes of the third-eye chakra mainly revolve around clarity versus confusion. When we already 'know', this is also because we fear confusion – anything that might destabilise our current structure of perception.

Learning how to remain open in a state of listening and receiving, while having a sufficient knowledge and capacity of discrimination, is the greatest challenge of the sixth chakra.

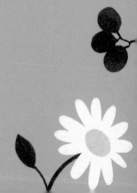

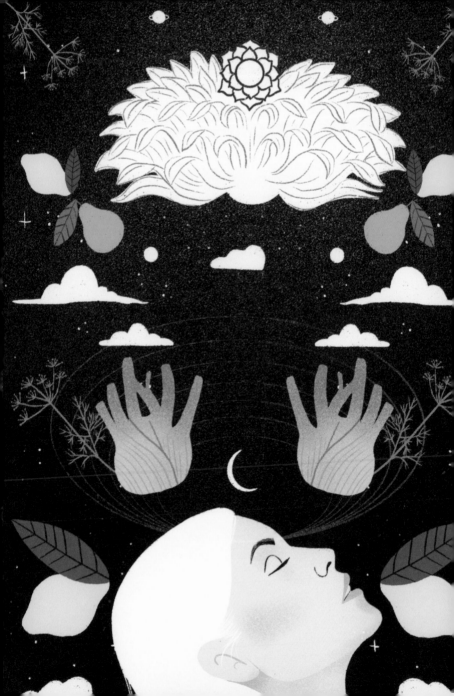

Crown Chakra
The Great White Light
Consciousness • Spirituality • Purity

Overview

Persona: Find your true north

Sanskrit name: *Sahasrara*

Meaning: Thousand fold

Colour: White/pearlescent or violet

Season: No associated season

Sense: Our thoughts

Element: Thoughts leading to understanding

Energy: Masculine

Psychological function: Understanding

Resulting in: Bliss

Identity: Universal identity

Qualities: Oneness, bliss, transcendence

Quest: The quest for returning to one's original spiritual nature and home. The quest for detachment from our earthly bondage and identification

Blocking fears: The death of the 'I-consciousness', leaving the world behind
Rights: To know and to learn
Challenge: Attachment
Location: Crown of the head
Associated symbol: A lotus with one thousand, or even infinite number of violet petals
Planet: Uranus
Body parts: Central nervous system, cerebral cortex and pineal gland

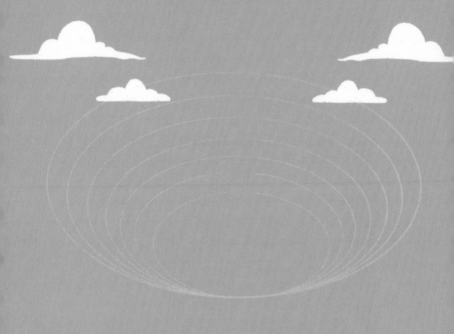

The balanced crown chakra

A person with a balanced and open crown chakra is fully aware that true bliss and happiness cannot be found in any of the experiences available for the ego here in this worldly existence of time and space, but rather, only in self-transcendence. They are uninterested in the possible satisfaction of worldly experiences and easily shift their attention, energy and ambition towards the realm of spiritual union, with the realisation that in diminishing the ego, real satisfaction is found.

In practice, they seek the type of knowledge that promotes non-attachment and deeper liberation from material objects. They are naturally inclined to meditation and silence, with meditation no longer feeling effortful. They have an ever-expanding sense of inner satisfaction that doesn't come from the external world, and so the incessant ego drive towards searching in the world significantly diminishes.

The imbalanced crown chakra

An imbalanced or blocked crown chakra is characterised by
an intense earthly gravity (due to imbalanced lower chakras),
resistance to the spiritual realm and the fear of losing a sense
of identity. The crown chakra energy becomes imbalanced
if there is a strong commitment towards maintaining
attachments to worldly possessions and engagements.

Another cause for a crown chakra imbalance is if a trauma took
place either in the spiritual realm or in an experience that is related
to an unexpected loss of boundaries of the self-consciousness.
A trauma may range from a powerful spiritual experience
(where they wished for some bliss and instead entered a
state of nothingness which scared them), or a sudden loss of
consciousness as in a near-death experience, surgery or a near-
fatal accident. All these incidents could cause an imprint upon
the crown chakra as a warning signal whenever we reach a similar
state of loss dissolution and opening to the infinite source of life.

Transcending the crown chakra

While the root chakra contains the more instinctual fear of the cessation of the body, the crown chakra holds a subtler fear: the very ending of the 'I-consciousness', the desire of continuity that our impermanent and perishable ego has.

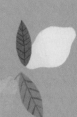

The crown chakra deals with deeper questions that strive to tap into the 'unknowable', as found in death and deep sleep. It invites us to experience states of self-transcendence in which our spirit is able to experience a great wholeness, and if we are able to transcend our ego's fear of death, there awaits a tremendous sense of liberation, oneness and bliss.

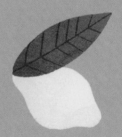

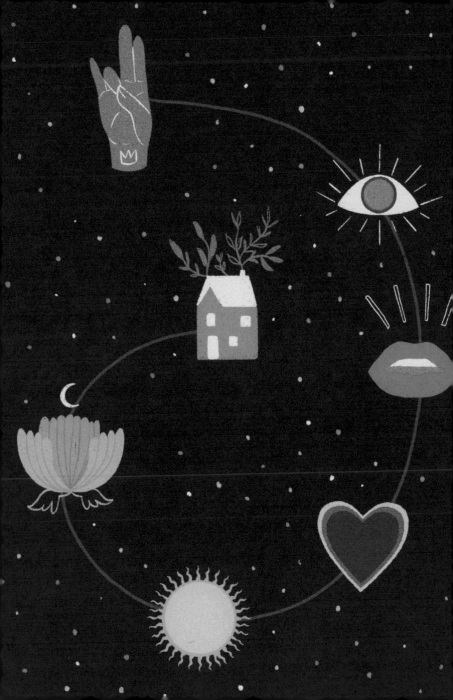

My Balance Superpowers

These seven balance superpowers are the basic needs I have identified for being your best self and aligning your chakras. If you can master and use these superpowers to your benefit, then you can achieve emotional clarity, a sense of balance and enhanced wellbeing, every day.

Using the lists provided for each chakra superpower, you should be able to work out which chakra(s) are over- or underactive. Armed with this and your understanding of each chakra as described in the previous chapter and how it relates to the energy in your life, you can work out which superpower you can use to bring about balance.

Start to follow my basic rebalancing rituals and cultivate and nurture them daily – it will soon feel like second nature to find support when you don't feel safe or trusting, to do something that lights your creative spark when life feels mundane and boring, or to use stillness when you feel the need to be in the moment.

Support • Creativity • Identity • Love• Truth • Intuition • Stillness

Support
Root chakra

As our instinctive centre, the root chakra deals with our basic needs and instincts, such as survival, fear and trust, and its main drive is to establish a solid sense of inner and outer security and stability. Its central question is 'Am I safe?'. The root chakra provides the entire system of mind, body and spirit with a sense of general wellbeing. It is the foundation of a well-sustained, nourished, solid and stable human being. Balancing the root chakra creates a solid foundation in which all chakras above are able to open and blossom.

It is one of my superpowers because when balanced, it offers you a tremendous amount of support through that sense of solid, stable ground beneath your feet. It makes you feel safe and secure in those moments of unease. It's for those moments in life when the rug gets pulled out from underneath your feet and you no longer know who or what you can trust and count on. This is when you most need support, and having a balanced root chakra will immediately help you determine exactly who and what you can rely on to offer you a helping hand and the support you need.

Utilising the root chakra as a superpower means connecting to what you associate as your 'home', be it a person (such as a parent or partner) or a physical place (like a country, the home you live in) or in a more spiritual context (you may describe your spiritual connection to something – such as religion – as your home). Your 'home' is where you feel you belong, where you fit in and can go to for support. It makes you feel safe and more rejuvenated than anything else on earth and is something you feel you can trust and depend on.

This superpower has the ability to build you up and really take care of you when you feel life is getting on top of you. When illness takes hold or major events happen that shake your very foundation (such as losing a job, moving countries or house, long-term relationship breakdowns, divorce, death of a loved one or natural disasters such as fire, flood, earthquakes, tsunamis, hurricanes, etc.), connecting to this superpower and utilising its ability to help you feel centred, safe and supported is essential when you feel imbalanced.

Underactive

- Burdened by life's daily tasks
- Clinginess, especially to family, for support
- Fixation on material possessions
- Diarrhoea
- Eating disorders
- Feeling vulnerable
- Paranoia
- Aggression
- Quick-temperedness
- Inability to relax
- A desire to control everything in their environment
- 'Control freak' personality

Balanced

- Healthy body
- Feeling safe and secure
- Independent
- Trusting
- Flexible
- Reliable
- Responsible
- Ability to relax and enjoy life
- Having a sense of belonging
- Fitting in easily within communities
- Strong tribal mentality
- Good family relationships
- Connected to your sense of home
- Feeling supported
- Having patience

Overactive

- Feeling disconnected from family
- Feeling overwhelmingly exhausted
- Tired more often than not
- Feelings of insecurity
- Feeling unsafe
- Feeling fearful or anxious
- Feeling unsupported
- Homesickness
- Financially unstable
- Worrying about basic needs such as money, food and shelter
- Feeling unmotivated
- Inability to focus
- Phobia to commitment
- Constipation
- Arthritis
- Knee and leg pain
- Sciatica

To balance your root chakra:

EAT

Red foods: tomatoes, raspberries, strawberries, hibiscus,
redcurrants

Root vegetables: beetroot, parsnips, carrots, sweet
potatoes, celeriac

Foods with a high soluble fibre content: chia and flaxseeds

Earthy-flavoured foods: mushrooms, cumin, beetroot, sage

Protein-rich foods: nuts and hummus, hemp seeds, spinach,

Vitamin D and calcium-rich foods for bone structure:
sesame seeds, tahini

Grounding spices: ginger, cinnamon, clove, nutmeg, cumin

Home-made, traditional foods, such as good old
'Mum's cooking' type of meals

Flavour combinations
Sweet potato and cinnamon
Beetroot and ginger
Carrot and cumin
Tomato and mushroom

ACT
Plant a garden
A wonderful way for you to balance and connect to your root
chakra is to place your hands in the earth. The very act of
putting a living organism's roots into soil or planting a seed
and helping it find stability and a place to call home can be
extremely nurturing to your root chakra.

If you don't have a garden, you could scatter some wildflower seeds into a public field. Or plant an indoor plant into a pot for your living room or herbs for your kitchen window ledge. If you have access to a small patch of earth, prune or nurture the plants already existing in the earth, or plant some new plants or seeds for the seasons ahead.

Define your 'home'
Each of us has a place on earth that resonates with us more than any other. This could be a physical place such as a country, county, house or holiday home. For some of us our 'home' could be with a specific person or with their family, and for others it could be a piece of furniture, a religion or faith, or even within themselves, as they find peace knowing their home is their centre or soul.

Your activity is to define what your home is. How it makes you feel, and why it feels safe and secure for you to go there and just be you. Write it down or visually walk around this place in your mind for at least 5 minutes in stillness while you feel every nook and cranny of this safe place for you.

Declutter your life
Let go of three items you no longer feel you identify with or no longer bring you joy. Recycle these items by taking them to a charity store or passing them onto someone who will use them and love as much as you once did.

Touch the earth
Take your shoes off where it is safe to do so outdoors and

go for a walk barefoot through a park or garden. Feel the earth between your toes and connect to the ground you stand on.

BE

Begin by taking a moment to sit and feel grounded in your seated position. Place your hands on your thighs, palms down, and begin breathing, deeply and slowly. Breathe audibly at first, and then allow your breathing to become increasingly quieter. Bring your awareness again to the weight of your seat and rise tall in your spine. Continue breathing evenly between the inhale and exhale until you feel present and steady at your core. Now ask yourself these questions (below) and allow yourself enough time before moving onto the next question to sit with your answer and analyse how the answers make you feel.

ASK

Who am I today? What three words would I use to define myself today?

Do I feel secure? Is there a sense of stability in my life today?

Do I feel safe? What would I need in order to feel even more safe today?

Where do I feel most at home? Where do I belong?

Who are the people in my 'tribe' whom I resonate with and want to connect with even more today?

Who or what do I trust in my life? Can I allow myself to let go and trust even more today?

What am I afraid of? Am I trying to control anything in my life that I no longer need to?

SAY

'I belong, my tribe understands and supports me.'
'I am eternally safe and I trust all that is around me.'
'I am grounded, centred and at peace.'
'I accept and nurture my body as it is.'
'I deserve abundance and prosperity.'

MOVE

Associated with the element earth, representing physical and emotional grounding, root chakra poses such as *tadasana*/mountain pose and *virabhadrasana*/warrior one often focus on the feet to help you feel grounded, as well as poses that stretch and strengthen the legs. These are designed to bring you back to your body, to the earth and the experience of safety, security and stillness.

When your hamstrings are tight, the contraction creates a sense that you're constantly prepared to run away. *Uttanasana*/standing forward bend and *janu sirsasana*/head-to-knee pose can help to create calmness, patience and a willingness to slow down and stay in one place. When you strengthen the quadriceps and open your hamstrings, you renew your confidence and commitment to the next steps in your life's journey. As you can lean into these poses and ease your fears, you may learn to trust the earth and your body.

Finishing your practice with peaceful restorative poses such as *supta baddha konasana*/reclining bound angle pose, *savasana*/corpse pose, and *balasana*/child's pose, all of which settle an overactive mind and encourage us to surrender to gravity. By the end of your practice, you will feel at home in your body and more prepared for the challenges that may await you in the day.

(Yoga is traditionally practised in the morning, but it can be done at any time of the day.)

SMELL
Use the following essential oils in your home or carry them with you sprinkled onto a handkerchief during the day: cedarwood, clove, ginger, myrrh and sandalwood. You can also dilute them in a carrier oil and massage into the soles of your feet and the base of your spine.

HOLD
Healing crystals: ruby, garnet, hematite – wear them in jewellery, place them under your pillow, or place them on your desk.

Creativity
Sacral chakra

The sacral chakra is associated with the element of water and is the home of your vitality because it regulates the flow of energy around your body. It is also responsible for your ability to create and enjoy life. Mastering it enables you to unlock pleasure and your deepest desires. It's hard to master but when you do, you release infinite energy and the ability to create what you truly want in life.

Utilising this chakra as a superpower means connecting to your creativity and everything that inspires and brings you joy (without going to excess). I am a huge fan of Brené Brown and her research into shame and vulnerability – she believes 'untapped creativity is not benign' and I agree with her. Creativity is the gateway to utilising this chakra as a superpower for times when life has started to zap your energy and nothing brings you pleasure any more.

When you stop having fun and become blinkered by your goals, this chakra is your antidote. Through it you can remind yourself that life doesn't have to be boring in the pursuit of goals and dreams. There must be room for your passions, having fun and being creative.

Underactive

- Lack of vitality
- Lack of creativity
- Depression
- Inability to feel joy or be playful
- Resisting change/fear of change
- Unable to go with the flow
- Lack of fun in life
- Reproductive disorders (painful periods, endometriosis, infertility or low libido)
- Urinary problems
- Kidney dysfunction

Balanced

- Vitality
- Boundless energy
- Creativity
- Passion
- Enthusiasm
- Individualism
- Spontaneity
- Flexibility and adaptability
- Feeling joy and excitement
- Able to have fun without inhibitions
- Feeling connected easily to others
- Maintaining many friendships

Overactive

- Living without any routine
- Craving variety
- Impatience
- Addictions
- Taking actions to the extreme

To balance your sacral chakra:

 ### EAT
Orange foods: papaya, mango, oranges, carrots, squash,
    sweet potatoes, apricots
Foods to improve absorption of nutrients and digestive
    health, such as fermented foods: miso, tempeh, kimchi,
    sauerkraut, kefir, kombucha, tamari, whole/live yoghurt
Foods for reproductive health: maca root powder, kelp
Cooking methods to help breakdown phylates: soaking,
    sprouting, choosing 'activated' foods and fermentation
Choose sourdough (fermented yeast) breads
Avoid refined sugars, high protein-rich foods and hard-
    to-digest foods

Flavour combinations
Carrot and orange
Squash and miso
Kimchi and kelp
Mango and yoghurt

 ### ACT
Create
Enjoy at least 30 minutes of creativity each day. This could
be through cooking, drawing, colouring, writing, gardening,
painting or photography. The objective is to allow self-
expression through something creative to help connect
you to yourself and your inner passions.

Get yourself out of the rut
At times when I feel life does feel a little 'stuck' or out of

balance, I like to get out my notepad and write at the top of the page 'I am looking forward to feeling....' And then I begin to list all the things that I am hoping and wishing I will feel that I may not be experiencing at the time. This process helps me to break down how I may achieve some of those feelings and see how I can adjust so that I am staying open to them being created in my life. Try it next time you feel like life needs a little more spice or you just don't seem to be feeling the way you want to on a daily basis.

Run to the water

The sacral chakra element is water, and a wonderful way to balance the sacral chakra is to go for a walk along a beach, have a bath, go for a swim or do something active in or on the water such as diving or kayaking. Or simply sit by a river, stream or waterfall and use the proximity to water to help balance your sacral chakra energy.

Dance

There is no better way to get the energy flowing in your body again than to move, and move in an enjoyable way. If your sacral chakra is imbalanced, the very thought of dancing may turn you right off, but trust me, try it.

Put some music on that will get your hips swaying, then slowly build from there. Either do it in the privacy of your own bedroom or go out and find others you can dance with – sometimes having others around who you can watch and move with you is all you need to get the momentum going... who knows, you may come home many hours later having had an absolute blast!

Enjoy a candlelit meal
Set the dining table beautifully and light some candles so you can melt into the evening with some soft music and delicious food. Have a date night in with your partner or family, or make it a solo date, honouring the relationship you have with yourself.

Glow from the inside out
Enjoy anything that makes you feel pampered and rejuvenated. If you don't have the time or money to head to your local day spa, then buy yourself some beautiful orange flowers such as tulips, roses, lilies, gerberas or daisies and place them in your home to bring you a sense of joy and rejuvenation every time you notice them.

BE
Begin by taking a moment to allow your belly to settle and feel relaxed. Place your hands on your navel area and begin bringing attention to your breath. Sense your belly opening and receiving the gentle wisdom of your emotional body with each breath. Allow your body to speak to itself and listen to what it needs today. Pay attention and honour the feelings as they cycle through your consciousness. These sensations are sacred messages of body intelligence, intended to keep you aware of what your body needs now. Now ask yourself these questions (below) and allow enough time before moving on to the next question to sit with your answer and analyse how your answers make you feel.

ASK
What is just one way I can feel excited and playful today? Do I allow myself to obsess or do things to excess in order

to find excitement or joy?

What is it that I don't allow myself to feel? Am I restricting or
    holding myself back from certain feelings?

Am I resisting change in my life? What am I trying to control?

Do aspects of my day-to-day life feel like a chore? If so, how
    can I make them feel more fun?

How can I be more creative today? How can I feel more joy?

What have I done recently that has felt adventurous? What
    adventures am I looking forward to going on soon?

SAY

'I am radiant, beautiful and strong, and enjoy a healthy
    and passionate life.'

'I flow when I release control.'

'I easily adapt to change.'

'I honour my desires and individuality.'

'I give myself permission to express my passion.'

MOVE

Along with the sacral chakra at the pelvis, the other even-
numbered chakras (the fourth, at the heart, and the sixth, at
the third eye) are connected with the 'feminine' energies of
relaxation and openness. These chakras exercise our rights
to feel, to love and to see. Odd-numbered chakras (found
in the legs and feet at the root chakra, solar plexus, throat,
and crown of the head) are connected with the 'masculine'
energies of applying our will on the world, asserting our
rights to have, to ask, to speak and to know.

Here in the feminine sacral chakra, asanas help us
with adaptability and receptivity. The leg position in
gomukhasana/cow face pose, forward bending with the legs

in the first stage of *eka pada rajakapotasana*/pigeon pose, *baddha konasana*/bound angle pose, *upavistha konasana*/ open angle pose, and other hip and groin openers all provide freedom of movement in the pelvis. These hip and groin openers should never be forced, for they require the subtle feminine touch of sensitivity and surrender.

Trikonasana/triangle pose, *bhujangasana*/cobra pose, *natarajasana*/dancer's or Shiva pose and *badhakonasana*/ butterfly pose are also great sacral chakra poses for inner confidence and healthy desires.

(Yoga is traditionally practised in the morning, but it can be done at any time of the day.)

SMELL
Use the following essential oils in your home or carry them with you sprinkled onto a handkerchief during the day: clary sage*, tangerine, rose geranium and patchouli. You can also dilute in a carrier oil and massage into the area slightly below the navel.
*Please note that clary sage essential oil should not be used during pregnancy.

HOLD
Healing crystals: coral, carnelian, yellow zircon – wear them in jewellery, place them under your pillow, or place them on your desk.

Identity
Solar plexus

While the first and second chakras are the main storehouses for our instincts, impulses and urges (such as seeking basic survival and pleasure), the solar plexus serves to answer the questions 'Who am I as a person and what do I want?' and 'What are my goals and dreams?'. Home of our will and power, it is our source of personal ambition and governs self-esteem, confidence, warrior energy and the power of transformation. Simply, it is your energy chakra, your powerhouse, where drive, ambition and willpower are allowed to thrive and propel us towards reaching our goals and dreams. The solar plexus also controls metabolism and digestion and fuels our bodies to feel energised and capable.

I love using this chakra as a superpower because, when balanced, it offers you your sense of identity and purpose on Earth. You feel strong, capable and powerful. You are buoyed by a sense of responsibility to your task and by a determination that allows you to feed your soul's purpose. You have a 'fire in your belly' and you wholeheartedly believe you are enough, what you do is enough; by staying true to who you are and what you want, you will succeed.

Although an amazing superpower for when we do need a little fire in our belly, we need to be careful not to allow this chakra to move into overdrive. With all the demands of a fast-paced westernised lifestyle where there are long work hours, demanding deadlines and financial debt, for some (mainly the alpha-type personality) the lure of power, success and everything they can bring means we leave ourselves vulnerable to being in *on*-mode all the time, glorifying that sense of being busy, in demand and working at a fast pace.

This superpower is for the overachiever who loves to feel busy and productive, who is never content with their own productivity and writes exhaustive lists of daily tasks, beating themselves up at the end of the day when they inevitably didn't cross every item off their list. They are constantly stressed and feel close to burnout, but prop themselves up with caffeine and other stimulants to keep energy high. Often this dogged approach towards their goals and dreams reflects the sense that they believe they are simply not enough and try to fill the void with achievements instead.

In juxtaposition to this, when the solar plexus is underactive the person may be prone to laziness. They feel unmotivated and love to procrastinate. They lack ambition and confidence and consequently often do the bare minimum to get by each day. Nurturing the solar plexus is essential for these people to find a sense of purpose and identity in this world so they are able to believe they are enough and feel empowered.

To tap into this superpower, you must first identify what sets you apart from anyone else. Ask yourself, 'Who am I?' and 'What gives me a sense of purpose?'. By identifying these important factors, you are then able to determine whether what you 'do' in your day-to-day life reflects this. If not, correcting this is your mission.

Underactive

- Low self-esteem
- Lacking in confidence
- No sense of purpose or direction
- Unmotivated
- Indecision
- Weakness
- Feeling of being powerless
- Laziness
- 'I am not enough' belief system
- Lack of personal boundaries
- Lack of self-respect
- No self-discipline
- Self-critical
- Fear of rejection
- Sluggish metabolism
- Skin and liver problems

Balanced

- Confidence
- High self-esteem
- Strong sense of self
- Purposeful
- Driven
- Ambitious
- Healthy determination
- Self-motivating
- Successful
- Self-disciplined
- Productive
- Decisive
- Can see a clear path forward
  to reach their goals
- Clarity in mind and actions
- Doing what you say you will do
- Strong willpower
- Good stress tolerance

Overactive

- Overweight
- Feeling highly stressed
- Constantly busy/need to feel busy
- A feeling of being 'wired' all the time
- Over-stimulated
- Working too hard
- Overwhelmed
- 'I am not enough' belief system
- Bossy
- Stubborn
- Need for control
- Chronic fatigue
- High blood pressure
- Blood-sugar imbalances

To balance your solar plexus:

EAT

Yellow foods: pineapple, bananas and passion fruit
Foods that offer the most 'fuel/energy' to our body
Complex carbohydrates: oats, beans and pulses of all kinds;
 legumes such as chickpeas, chestnuts, corn/popcorn,
 sweet potatoes, squash
Fruits and sweeteners: bananas, honey, dates, prunes,
 molasses
Adaptogenic and tonic herbs: lucuma, licorice, turmeric
B vitamin-rich foods to boost metabolism: nutritional yeast
Avoid stimulating foods such as caffeine – can be too
 stimulating for the overactive solar plexus

Flavour combinations

Pineapple and passion fruit
Banana and dates
Turmeric and chickpeas
Oats and honey

ACT
Build a fire

Being around fire is a wonderful way for you to balance
your solar plexus. Either have a bonfire in the garden or, if
you have one, light the open fire in your home. If this is not
possible, light a candle and focus on the flickering flame.

Eat that frog!

Think of something you have been putting off for a while.
Think about why you have been putting it off and write down
five steps you can take to begin working towards this goal.

Manage that to-do list

If you have a to-do list, take a new piece of paper and draw a line down the middle of the page. On the left-hand side, write down everything that is on your to-do list – the full exhaustive list – and then in the right-hand column, choose one to three things you can realistically complete in the next 24 hours. This will prevent overwhelm and allow you to feel productive with your time by being able to see a completed list for the day. Do the same thing tomorrow, making sure to manage both lists and make sure they are achievable.

Get familiar with your non-negotiable list

List between seven and ten things you know you need that are non-negotiable in your day-to-day life in order to feel balanced, such as drinking water, getting at least seven hours' sleep, connecting to loved ones, meditation, going to the gym, taking your supplements or going for a walk.

Be spontaneous and try something new

This doesn't have to be major – even experiences like trying a different restaurant, going into a new shop, visiting a new park or checking out a local art exhibition can shake up the energy and bring healing to your solar plexus.

Breathing exercise

Improve both digestion and metabolism with the *bhastrika* breath, ideally in the morning. It may take time to get used to, but once you do you will enjoy the fire it builds within you. Sit comfortably with the spine tall and shoulders relaxed. Start taking a few deep breaths in and out of the nose with the lips closed. Then, forcefully inhale through the nose while inflating the lower abdomen and forcefully exhale through the nose while pressing the lower abdomen towards the spine. Use one-half count on the inhalation and one-half count on the exhalation at a rapid pace. You will feel like you're getting an abdominal workout. Try for ten repetitions then work up to 15 or 20. After you're finished, you will feel a tingling or glowing feeling around the navel.

 ## BE

Begin by taking time to sit quietly, hands on your thighs, palms up, arms straight and relaxed, index fingers and thumbs touching. Allow your spine to rise tall to create a sense of readiness. Let your breathing rise and fall naturally, bringing awareness to the space just below your heart. Notice it feeling energised and filled with warming energy. Feel confidence rise within you as you ask these questions (below). Allow enough time before moving on to the next question to analyse how the answers make you feel.

 ## ASK

How does my energy feel today? Do I feel vibrant, radiant?
What am I striving for today? Are my tasks exciting, motivating?
Are my goals and dreams achievable? Do I have a clear path towards reaching them?
Is there anything I am avoiding or procrastinating over?
What external expectations do I currently feel?
Have I said the words 'I should…' in the last few months? If so, how can I change that into 'I will…'?

 ## SAY

'I accept myself completely. I accept that I have strengths and I accept that I have weaknesses.'
'My boundaries are respected and upheld.'

'I am enough' or 'I am worthy.'

'There is a deep sense of motivation inside me.'

'My existence is powerful.'

'I know what I want and have the energy and will to go out and manifest it easily.'

'My potential is unlimited.'

'I am responsible for what I create.'

 ## MOVE

Solar plexus poses fan the flames of our inner fire and restore vitality. Practise *surya namaskar*/sun salutations, abdominal strengtheners like *navasana*/boat pose, *ardha navasana*/half boat pose, and *urdhva prasarita padasana*/leg lifts, warrior poses and twists. Restorative, passive backbends like *setu bandhasana*/bridge pose can be calming agents for the third chakra if the energy here is excessive.

(Yoga is traditionally practised in the morning, but it can be done at any time of the day.)

 ## SMELL

Use the following essential oils in your home or carry them with you sprinkled onto a handkerchief during the day: lemon, citronella*, lemongrass, fennel and juniper*. You can also dilute in a carrier oil and massage into the area between the navel and the ribcage.

*Please note that citronella and juniper essential oils should not be used during pregnancy.

 ## HOLD

Healing crystals: amber, topaz, apatite – wear them in jewellery, place them under your pillow, or place them on your desk.

Love
Heart chakra

The fourth chakra, also referred to as the heart chakra, is literally at the heart of it all! To me, this is the most important chakra as it sits perfectly at the centre of the seven chakras with three below and three above. This is where the physical energies from the three lower chakras unite with the spiritual energies of the three chakras above the heart; where the physical stability and trust you've built for yourself, along with your vitality, passions and sense of identity, marry with your visionary mind, your authentic voice and intuition – allowing you to fully express and open your heart's true desire and live a life with unconditional love, compassion, forgiveness and gratitude every day.

Love *is* your ultimate superpower because if you master and balance this chakra successfully, then you are able to give and receive love to and from others, unconditionally! But most importantly, you open the door to fully love yourself without expectation or judgement.

I use this superpower in *everything* I do – it's the 'mode' I choose to see and assess the world from. I use it when I need to accept something that I did not choose or expect, when pain, grief, hurt and betrayal come knocking, in those moments of compromise that happen from time to time. I use it when something just isn't 'sitting right' within me and I need to reconcile with it and for all the moments in life that make you question if this is right for you. It can simply be when negative energy comes your way and life feels like a struggle.

Before I speak, before I allow my mind to start making decisions and especially before I let my ego get involved, I use the power of love and gratitude as my language and compass to allow me to assess and to guide me. If I choose to only see the world through the lens of love and gratitude, then I never allow anger, resentment or frustration to guide and influence me.

Being able to utilise this chakra as a superpower requires you to see all living things as connected through the power of love, to find the ability to be kind in everything you do, to yourself and all others. This is the truest test of life and your mission here in the heart chakra.

Underactive

- Struggling to accept life's circumstances
- Heartache
- Grief
- Anger
- Fear of betrayal or abandonment
- Hatred towards others and yourself
- Problematic or draining relationships
- Disconnection in relationships
- Shyness
- Lack of empathy
- Judgement
- Needing validation for fulfilment
- Low self-esteem
- Defensiveness
- Distrust
- Possessiveness
- Highly critical of others
- Asthma
- Heart and lung disease

Balanced

- Loving
- Grateful
- Compassionate
- Forgiving
- Accepting others and yourself
- Is able to maintain intimate relationships
- Having healthy personal boundaries
- Trusting
- Non-judgemental
- Kind
- Empathetic
- Able to let go of the past
- Gives love unconditionally
- Can see love in everything

Overactive

- Anger
- Jealousy
- Co-dependency
- Fear of loneliness
- Constantly doing things for others
- Using money to show affection
- Constantly needing comfort from others

To balance your heart chakra:

 EAT

Green foods: broccoli, green herbs, asparagus, courgettes (zucchini), cucumber, lettuce, edamame, peas, green beans

Offer your body the most potent phyto-nutrient-dense foods: spirulina, moringa, wheatgrass, barley grass

Leafy-green vegetables: kale, spinach, chard and rocket (arugula)

Healthy fats: avocados, nuts, seeds

Preparation methods: juicing and smoothies for quick absorption of nutrients

Food made with love, such as meals made for sharing: mezze, tapas, antipasti

Avoid stimulating foods: caffeine, refined sugars

Flavour combinations

Courgette (zucchini) and basil

Asparagus and tarragon

Pea and mint

Avocado and coriander (cilantro)

 ACT

Love, love, love

Simply put, give love. Find a way to express your love to the people in your life, whether it's with physical touch, like a hug or a kiss, a thoughtful gift, words of gratitude, or some other means that feels good to you and they appreciate and understand as an offering of your love.

Begin each day with a grateful heart

Write down all the things you are grateful for today. Start with the simplest things, such as your lungs for allowing you to breathe, your heart for allowing you to pump blood around your body, and the life you were gifted by your mother and father bringing you into this life. Start to add other things you are grateful for around these. Include people and things that enable you to live your life every day.

Fall in love with yourself

Practise loving yourself. Take note of harsh thoughts and feelings that your mind directs at you. Notice them, acknowledge them and then let them go. You can build up to replacing them with kind and loving thoughts and feelings. If it helps, write down the kind and loving thoughts and feelings and leave them somewhere you will see them daily.

The act of giving

A great way to feel grateful for what we have is to start giving. Why not try to find a way to put the act of giving into motion? Try a random act of kindness, offer your time or simply hug someone who needs it. Give it a go; you've got absolutely nothing to lose and everything to gain!

Forgive

Life gives us opportunities to feel pain, hurt and disappointment from those around us all the time. Give yourself permission to let go of a grievance you have been holding onto and truly forgive that person. Send them love and be grateful for how that pain, hurt or disappointment has helped you grow and develop.

Breathing exercise

Stand with your arms by your sides. Exhale through your nose, emptying your lungs completely (ideally, all inhales and exhales should be through your nose). Immediately inhale deeply through your nose and as you inhale, slowly bring your arms over your head and bring your palms to touch, then pull up on your toes, raising your heels as far off the ground as possible. Hold the breath for the count of five. Slowly exhale fully through your nose, until all the breath has been released from your body. At the same time, slowly lower your arms by your sides and place your heels on the ground again. Hold the breath for the count of five. Repeat the exercise ten times, without pause.

 ## BE

Find a comfortable position where your back is fully supported. Try lying down completely or with your feet up a wall, or sitting in a chair or on the floor with your back against the wall. Once you have found your place, pay attention to your breath. Notice your body: where is there spaciousness? Where is there tension? Move your attention to your back and its contact with the chair, wall or floor. Allow yourself to feel supported. Holding this support in your body's awareness, turn your breath and attention towards your heart space. Is there fear? Is there hope? Is there a bit of both? Just notice. Once again, release into the support against your back as deeply as you are able. As you do, is there room to relax and soften your heart space? And to create more space on the exhale? Explore without judgement. When you are ready, begin to expand your attention to the room around you, feeling only love for everything around you. Now ask yourself these questions (below) and allow yourself enough time before moving on to the next question to sit with your answer and analyse how the answers make you feel.

ASK

Am I kind in my interactions with others?

Do I give love and connection without the need for a reward?

Are any of my relationships only or heavily biased towards what I can get from the relationship?

Is there anyone I need to forgive?

Do I feel worthy of love today?

What are three things I am grateful for today?

What expectations am I holding onto for others and myself?

SAY

'I am worthy of love.'

'I am kind to myself and others.'

'Love is my guiding truth in life and I give and receive love effortlessly and unconditionally.'

'I act from love.'

'I am able to let go of hurt and forgive myself and others with compassion.'

'I am grateful.'

MOVE

Asanas that lift and balance the energy within the heart chakra include passive chest openers in which you arch gently over a blanket or bolster, shoulder stretches such as the arm positions of *gomukhasana*/cow face pose and *garudasana*/eagle pose, and backbends such as *marjariasana*/cat pose and *ustrasana*/camel pose. Being an even-numbered, feminine chakra, the heart centre naturally yearns to release and let go. Doing backbends develops the trust and surrender we need to open the heart fully.

When we feel fearful, there is no room for love, and our bodies show constriction. When we choose love, the fear melts away, and our practice takes on a joyful quality. In many backbend poses, the heart is positioned higher than the head. It's wonderfully refreshing to let the mind drop away from the top position and instead lead with the heart.

Signs that this chakra is imbalanced include co-dependency, possessiveness, jealousy, heart disease and high blood pressure. For these symptoms, forward bends such as *uttanasana*/forward bending pose are the best antidote, because they are grounding and foster introspection.

(Yoga is traditionally practised in the morning, but it can be done at any time of the day.)

 ## SMELL
Use the following essential oils in your home or carry them with you sprinkled onto a handkerchief during the day: rose, jasmine and laurel*. You can also dilute in a carrier oil and massage into the chest and heart area.
*Please note that laurel essential oil should not be used during pregnancy.

 ## HOLD
Healing crystals: emerald, tourmaline, jade – wear them in jewellery, place them under your pillow, or place them on your desk.

Truth
Throat chakra

In my experience, this is the chakra most people struggle to master, but it is the most liberating superpower by far! To live an authentic life, wholeheartedly, in lifestyle, speech and through every level of self-expression is, to me, pure freedom. Home of our creative self-expression, communication with the world and authentic identity, to open and balance this chakra enables you to speak, listen and express your absolute, purest truth. Now isn't that a real superpower in this day and age?

Too often in today's society we fulfil the ambitions of our loved ones, shying away from doing what we truly want to do and be for fear of judgement or negative consequences. When there is conflict between what our heart desires and what our brain perceives to be the right thing to do or say, the throat chakra gets caught in the middle, literally, and our truth can often be ignored, silenced, pushed aside or swallowed and never allowed to be heard out of fear, guilt, shame or pride.

That's why mastering this chakra and using truth as a superpower in your everyday life is so important. However, the work doesn't start here in the throat chakra alone; this chakra requires the first and second chakras (the root and the sacral chakras) to have processed and overcome fear. The solar plexus needs to be confident and clear in its direction and path towards personal ambition and power, and the heart chakra needs to know what the heart desires and to have accepted the past. Only then can true expression be communicated through our needs, desires and opinions. If the lower chakras are aligned, then the throat chakra can fully open and discover how to be honest to oneself and the world around us.

Underactive

- Tight shoulders
- Silence – not wanting to speak
- A 'person of few words'
- Fear of being powerless
- Lying
- Shyness
- Lack of focus on the topic being discussed
- Not wanting to engage in conversation
- Scared of saying the wrong thing
- Scared of being judged
- Recurring sore throat
- Underactive thyroid
- Neck pain
- Dental pain

Balanced

- Able to speak your truth
- Effective communicator
- Good listener
- Influential
- Honest
- Trustworthy
- Authentic in everything you do and say
- Freely expressing your creative pursuits
- Liberated by your inner voice
- Loves to sing
- Good at public speaking
- Express yourself clearly and articulately
- At peace with your inner and outer worlds

Overactive

- Being overly talkative – the 'chatterbox'
- Frequently interrupting others during conversations
- Lying
- Gossiping
- Manipulating what you heard others say
- Compulsive eating
- Overactive thyroid
- Tension in the jaw
- Teeth grinding at night

To balance your throat chakra:

EAT
Blue-hued foods: blueberries, raisins, cranberries, plums, rhubarb

Herbs to help the throat and thyroid: sage, elderberries, echinacea, manuka honey, ginger

Broths and foods to help you feel better when you are ill: ginger and garlic

Immune-boosting vitamin C-rich foods: strawberries, parsley, kiwi fruit, goji berries

Iodine-rich foods: kelp and sunflower seeds

Avoidance of stimulating foods: caffeine, refined sugars

Flavour combinations
Blueberry and goji berry

Plum and raisin

Sage and rhubarb

Cranberry and ginger

ACT
Sing from the rooftops
Sing! Singing is an amazing throat chakra cleanser, so sing your favourite song out loud and enjoy opening up your voice to those high notes.

Enjoy a vocal massage
This is a kind of massage that focuses on releasing the muscles around your neck and jaw. This kind of massage is great for loosening up those vocal cords in readiness for the moment we are ready to speak our truth. You will need to find a specialised practitioner to do this.

Take note of your subconscious mind

Start keeping a dream journal. When you aren't doing a great job of expressing yourself during your waking hours, your spirit sometimes tries to express itself in dreams. Writing them down helps you to pay attention to the messages and hopefully gain some clarity about how to speak your truth and move in the direction of your higher self. Regularly review your journal. Try reading recent passages out loud – this is a great way for you to assess if what your voice says feels congruent within your body.

Write a letter

If you don't yet feel ready to speak your truth, then writing a letter can be a great way for you to express it via a note addressed to the person you would like to tell your truth to. Whether you send the letter or not is irrelevant, as the process of writing can be cathartic enough.

Cultivate the skill of listening

Find someone to listen to. Give yourself over to fully listening to them for five minutes. Do this without making comments – including non-verbal gestures. Then switch and have them do the same for you. Talk about whatever is on your mind. When both of you are finished, neither should comment on what the other said. Just thank each other for sharing and listening.

 ## BE

Take a cleansing breath in and breathe out the tension in your body. Allow your breathing to fall into its own natural rhythm, not trying to control it in any way. Just observe as you breathe in relaxation, and breathe out tension. Bring your attention to your throat area. Imagine a lovely little sky-blue light there, swirling around like a little whirlpool. Try to notice how it feels, how it looks. Try to get a sense of how it is functioning – can you feel any tingling? Is it swirling and moving, what speed is it, does it feel fast or slow, a little small light or a big enlarged light? What thoughts are popping into your head? As you focus on this spinning blue wheel, focus on your truest expressions and ask yourself these questions (below), allowing yourself enough time before moving on to the next question to sit with your answer and analyse how the answers make you feel.

 ## ASK

Do I speak what is in my heart freely, openly and truthfully?
Do I express myself authentically through my words?
Do I feel listened to by those around me?
Do I hold back from speaking my truth? When?
What do I need to say that I haven't said out loud yet?
What don't I feel comfortable expressing yet? Why?

 ## SAY

'I live and communicate my truth.'
'I follow my passions in order to honour my purpose.'
'My voice matters.'
'I am honest and value honesty in others.'
'I fully express myself.'
'I listen and observe everything that is around me.'
'When I speak, I do not back away from what is true.'

 ## MOVE

The throat chakra resonates with our inner truth and helps us find a personal way to convey our voice to the outside world. The rhythm of music, the creativity of dance, the vibration of singing, and the communication we make through writing and speaking are all fifth chakra ways to express ourselves. During this practice I like to turn some music on and enjoy singing along and having a boogie.

Deficient energy in this chakra leads to neck stiffness, shoulder tension, teeth grinding, throat ailments and possibly an underactive thyroid. Excessive talking, an inability to listen, hearing difficulties, stuttering and an overactive thyroid are all related to excessiveness in this chakra. Depending on the ailments, different neck stretches and shoulder openers, including *ustrasana*/camel pose, *setu bandha sarvangasana*/bridge pose, *sarvangasana*/shoulder stand and *halasana*/plough pose, can all aid the fifth chakra.

(Yoga is traditionally practised in the morning, but it can be done at any time of the day.)

SMELL
Use the following essential oils in your home or carry them with you sprinkled onto a handkerchief during the day: Roman and German chamomile, bergamot, peppermint and wintergreen. You can also dilute in a carrier oil and massage into the throat area.

HOLD
Healing crystal: turquoise – wear it in jewellery, place it under your pillow, or place it on your desk.

Intuition
Third-eye chakra

Call it your gut feeling, natural instincts, your perception, inner knowing, intuition or simply a hunch, this superpower is about utilising the part of you that has the ability to understand something instinctively without the need for conscious reasoning.

This superpower is essential for a balanced life as it allows us to develop trust and confidence in ourselves. We can trust our decisions to perceive things as they really are and to feel confident in our awareness of the world around us. Instead of viewing the world as a series of events or observing our bodies through signs and symptoms, when we open the third eye we can see how the world functions as a whole and interpret what our body needs in order to be healthy. We become wise and our wisdom guides us.

When we master this superpower we are able to live in reality with clarity and insight, but also transcend it and open our conscious mind to visualise and imagine. Thus to open the third eye is to embrace our ability to 'see' what is right for us, what we need, our future and how everything is interconnected in our physical world.

Underactive

- Depression
- Never remember dreams
- Foggy, tired and indecisive state of mind
- Disorientation
- Disconnected
- Numbness
- Procrastination
- Forgetfulness/poor memory
- Inability to see a clear vision or goal to work towards
- Difficulty seeing patterns
- Inability to visualise
- Lack of imagination
- Hearing loss
- Hormone dysfunction and imbalances
- Eye strain

Balanced

- Vivid imagination
- Clarity
- Easily remember dreams
- Considered wise
- Intuitive
- Perceptive
- Psychic
- Able to trust your gut instincts
- Able to see 'the bigger picture'

Overactive

- Nightmares
- Insomnia
- Anxiety
- A constantly busy mind
- Headaches
- Hallucinations
- Sinus problems
- Inability to focus and concentrate
- Exaggerated imagination
- Hormone dysfunction and imbalances
- Mood swings
- Volatility

To balance your third eye:

EAT
Purple foods: blackberries, red cabbage, grapes, radicchio,
   balsamic vinegar, figs, olives
Brain-stimulating foods: matcha, cacao, coffee
Calming foods to the mind: chamomile, lavender, lemon
   verbena
Avoidance of stimulating foods: caffeine, refined sugars

Flavour combinations
Radicchio and olives
Balsamic vinegar and figs
Blackberry and chamomile
Coffee and chocolate

ACT
Invest in visualisation
Imagine a goal you would like to achieve, then find a
comfortable place to sit and begin to visualise what it would
feel like to wake up in your body once you have reached that
goal. Walk around in your life as if you are living the life you
imagine with your goals and dreams realised.
Or
Imagine your life in three to five years from now. What will
your body look like? Who will be in your life? Where will
you be living? How will you be spending your time? Try to
visualise every detail of your future life with as few barriers
as possible to the life you could be living – allow yourself to
fully express your deepest desires for your future.

Now allow yourself to feel the emotions you will experience if you live this life and achieve these goals and dreams.

Keep a dream journal

As a way of tapping into your unconscious mind, write down as much as you can remember about your dreams.

Star gaze on a clear night

Staring into the universe that exists around us can open our minds to the much larger picture we live in and are part of.

Cultivate a dialogue with the Divine

Ask a question and then relax into waiting for a response. Remember the Divine speaks to us in messages, signs and symbols. Be prepared to wait and be open to receiving information in any form. Look for moments in your life that feel serendipitous or like a strange coincidence. These can often reveal patterns and guidance, which can be beneficial.

Tame the monkey mind

The constant chatter of the mind is often referred to as the monkey mind. It jumps up and down, left and right, without notice and takes us everywhere with it. The monkey mind is seductive and appealing, it is untamed and does what it wants. A thought here, another one there, mixing together the story, then another thought, an emotion, a reaction and the story gets bigger and stronger – a monkey mind is constantly busy and relentlessly scatty. With practice you can learn to tame this monkey mind. The first step is to begin noticing when the monkey mind has taken over. Attempt to train your mind to catch the monkey mind out and when you do catch it, don't judge yourself. Just take a few deep breaths and let the chatter go and recentre your thoughts.

Yoga can help tame the monkey mind; it can bring truth by helping you to observe, then to let go of the habits you cling to and the stories you use to protect yourself. As you practise, you become intimate with your body, which many of us spend a lifetime either alienated from or waging war with. Yoga practice can pierce emotional places that most of us guard or avoid. Our bodies are intelligent – they are more a source of direct truth than our minds, but rarely do we listen to the wisdom that's buried in our beautiful chambers.

BE

Begin to tune into your intuitive power, your ability to perceive, know and experience with all your senses beyond the realm of the physical and into the realm of the divine. Breathe deeply into your lower abdomen, letting it fill up with the light of the Divine that is all around you. Breathe in and breathe out. As you exhale, let go of any tension, worry or struggle, any energy which is not yours. Breathe in the Divine light that is all around you and as you breathe out, feel yourself relaxing deeply, entering fully into this present space and time, becoming aware and becoming present.

Focus on your breath, and as you take in another deep breath through your nose, now breathe air into your lower abdomen, filling yourself up with light of the Divine. Now as you exhale, tune into your energetic field, which is infused with the Divine light all around you. Imagine your energy as a sort of hourglass shape, receiving with open arms the light of the Divine, intuitive guidance, infinite wisdom, wellbeing, healing and love, which flow down into your being from above. Imagine the middle of your hourglass energetic form being strong, stable and present.

Your core of energy is filled with light, helping you to increase your awareness, be fully present at this time, then flowing out and down, grounding you to the earth. Light flows down to the core of earth where you are able to feel your oneness with the Divine through earth with all that is. Now ask yourself these questions (below) and allow yourself enough time before moving on to the next question to sit with your answer and analyse how the answers make you feel.

ASK

Do I trust myself today?

What do I intuit about myself today?

Do I remember my dreams from last night's sleep?

What do I need to spend some time reflecting on?

Does my mind feel clear and focused today? If not, what is creating the fog?

What do I refuse to see?

SAY

'I am aware of the wisdom that dwells within me and I am in tune with it.'

'I am connected to my higher self and I honour and follow my intuition.'

'I think clearly and trust my decisions.'

'I visualise all that I want to create for myself and the world that I live in.'

'I am open to new perspectives.'

'I am present, I am mindful, I am here.'

MOVE

Poses that support the third-eye chakra are supported forward bends, adding an extra bolster or blanket to press upon and stimulate the third-eye area, or simply drop into *balasana*/child's pose and rest your forehead upon your mat.

Other poses to help connect to your inner voice include *adho mukha svanasana*/downward facing dog, *vajrasan*/thunderbolt pose and *anjaneyasana*/low lunge pose.

(Yoga is traditionally practised in the morning, but it can be done at any time of the day.)

 ## SMELL

Use the following essential oils in your home or carry them with you sprinkled onto a handkerchief during the day: rosemary, oregano, thyme* and linden. You can also dilute in a carrier oil and massage into the area between the eyebrows.
*Please note that thyme essential oil should not be used during pregnancy.

 ## HOLD

Healing crystals: quartz, lapis – wear them in jewellery, place them under your pillow, or place them on your desk.

Stillness
Crown chakra

In an age of distraction nothing can feel more luxurious than paying attention. Where there is constant movement, nothing is more important than sitting still. Often we are happiest when we forget time and just allow our minds to wander. The 'way of the crown chakra' is stillness, otherwise known as meditation, a superpower designed to allow you to find presence and a state where all is pure, simple and intentional. In this state, our minds are free to detach from the ego and live in the blissful present moment.

The crown chakra is the home of our enlightenment and spiritual connection to all that is. It opens a connection to our higher selves, to every being on the planet, and ultimately the Divine energy that creates everything in the universe – practising stillness unlocks this chakra and offers the rewards of serenity, joy and deep peace.

In essence, stillness is often more about cultivating the skill of listening than the quietening of our minds. Honouring our inner consciousness by paying attention to thoughts as they come and go is the process of stillness.

Underactive

- Frustration with life
- Spiritual scepticism
- Lack of purpose
- Depression
- Mental fog
- Fear of alienation
- Poor and inconsistent
  sleep patterns
- Confusion
- Apathy
- Materialism

Balanced

- Deep empathy for others
- Deep connection to the divine
- Aware of your divine purpose
- Clarity on all levels
- Expressing and sharing unconditional love
- Practising mindfulness
- Stillness
- Sense that you are being watched over
- Can easily meditate
- Allowing thoughts to come and go freely
- Able to detach from material objects
- Living without the need for the ego

Overactive

- Confusion
- Isolation
- Self-destructive behaviours
- Headaches
- Excess worry
- Nightmares
- Fatigue
- Frustration
- Boredom
- Greed/materialism
- Spiritual or intellectual elitism
- Entitlement
- Loneliness
- Anger
- Sensitivity to light and sound
- Rigid thoughts

To balance your crown chakra:

 ## EAT

When choosing foods for this chakra you should focus more on fasting and detoxing than the kind of foods used to build and maintain your body's strength and stamina.

White foods: fennel, pears, cauliflower, radishes, coconut

Light, very easy to digest food: sprouts, grapefruit, lemons, limes, pomelo

Mostly liquids: teas, juices, broths, healthy ice lollies

Detoxifying foods: lemons, grapefruit, avocados, artichokes

Small portions.

Avoidance of dense, heavy foods.

Flavour combinations
Fennel and lemon
Pear and fennel
Grapefruit and radish
Pomelo, coconut and lime

 ## ACT
Become aware

This exercise is incredibly powerful because it helps us notice and appreciate simple elements of our environment in a more profound way. It is designed to connect us with the beauty of the natural environment, something that is easily missed when we are rushing around in our busy lives.

1. Choose a natural object from within your immediate environment and focus on watching it for a minute or two. This could be a tree, flower or an insect, or even the clouds or the moon.

2. Don't do anything except notice the thing you are looking at. Simply relax into watching for as long as your concentration allows.
3. Look at this object as if you are seeing it for the first time. Visually explore every aspect of its formation, and allow yourself to be consumed by its presence. Allow yourself to connect with its energy and its purpose within the natural world.
4. Ask yourself if you feel connected to this object in some way.

Practise stillness

Sit in silence (with your eyes open or closed). Try to disconnect from the world around you for between 1–10 minutes every time you need to reconnect to the present moment. Put away your devices and sit, observing what thoughts come and go and any discomfort you might feel.

Learn how to live in service

Look for ways to practise selfless service. Helping others is a perfect way to feel compassion and oneness with humanity. Remember that all the great spiritual masters practised serving others – why not try volunteering or simply do an act of kindness for someone who really needs a little help.

BE

Take a cleansing breath in and breathe out the tension in your body. Allow your breathing to fall into its own natural rhythm, not trying to control it in any way. Just observe as you breathe in relaxation, and breathe out tension. Imagine a big, white lotus flower with its petals closed in the same place as your crown chakra. Look at the lotus and contemplate its shape, colour and texture. As you pay attention, the lotus slowly starts to swirl along with the chakra. One by one the petals of the lotus start to open.

As the first layer flowers, you see uncountable rows of more petals still to open. With every new petal opening the lotus starts spinning faster. You realise that every such opening leads to yet another layer of closed petals. The blooming of the lotus is an ongoing process of infinite stages. Now see your seventh chakra spinning with equal strength.

The chakra's violet light washes over you and pervades every cell, every pore in your body. Breathe deeply and feel the energy from your crown chakra connecting you to the sky above and the earth below, and everything in between, so you become one with existence. Rest in this awareness, then ask yourself these questions (below) and allow enough time before moving on to the next question to sit with your answer and analyse how the answers make you feel.

 ### ASK
Do I see everything around me as one?
Can I transcend my ego today?
Can I offer unconditional love to everything around me?
What do I choose to believe in?
What am I attached to or choose to hold onto in this world?
Do I know my higher purpose here on this earth?
I choose to believe the universe is....?

 ### SAY
'I am divine.'
'I have a divine purpose and I am deeply fulfilled in all that

I do.'
'I trust in infinite possibilities.'
'I go beyond my limiting beliefs and accept myself fully.'
'I feel connected to all living beings.'
'I am one with the universe.'

 ## MOVE

Meditation is the yogic practice best suited for bringing this chakra into balance, thus *padmasana*/lotus pose is expected here. The energy of this chakra helps us to experience the Divine, to open to a higher or deeper power, allowing the mind to become more present, clear and insightful.

Poses to help you connect to this pose include *sirsasana*/headstand pose, *matsyasana*/fish pose and *vriksasana*/tree pose.

(Yoga is traditionally practised in the morning, but it can be done at any time of the day.)

 ## SMELL

Use the following essential oils in your home or carry them with you sprinkled onto a handkerchief during the day: frankincense, angelica* and lavender. You can also dilute in a carrier oil and massage into the top of the head.
*Please note that angelica essential oil should not be used during pregnancy.

 ## HOLD

Healing crystals: diamond, amethyst – wear them in jewellery, place them under your pillow, or place them on your desk.

Your Everyday Balance Toolkit

Of all the pages in this book, the next few are the ones you need to bookmark. These four steps are your everyday balance toolkit – think of them as your coping strategy and for those times when life gives you a nudge and throws you off balance.

When you find yourself in a situation that is overwhelming, is causing you stress or burden, these four steps will help you rebalance and find your centre again so you can move forward in a considered and conscious manner.

Follow these four steps as many times as you need to until you start to feel centred and at peace again. Over time they will become instinctual, and balance will seem easy to invite into your everyday.

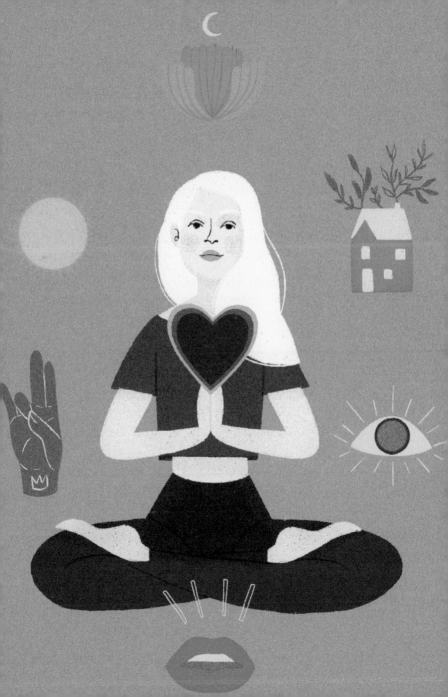

LOVE

Step 1

Your first step towards balance is to open your heart and allow gratitude to flood your mind. There is always something we can find to be grateful for and this is a great way to start to deal with any problem. Engaging your heart means you will make a decision from a place of compassion and acceptance.

Ask yourself:
What can I be grateful for in this situation or in this very moment?
What do I need to accept?
Who do I need to shower with compassion?

IDENTITY and TRUTH

Step 2

Your second step towards balance is to check in with your sense of identity.

Ask yourself:
Does this situation allow me to feel empowered and aligned morally and ethically?
What do I need in this moment in order to maintain congruency in who I am as a person, what I believe in and what I stand for?
How can I turn this situation into a positive experience where I feel energised and powerful?

Once you've checked in with your identity, it's time to speak your truth. Clear, authentic expression is key to allow clarity in any situation.

CREATIVITY and INTUITION

Step 3

Once you've found clarity and checked that your heart and identity are aligned, it's time to listen to your intuition. Tune in and listen to that 'gut feeling'. What is it saying to you? Are you getting signals that could help you get even more clarity and perspective here?

If your intuition tells you you are on the right path, it's time to allow the energy to flow and find its new equilibrium. Remember, life is not static – we are dynamic human beings and our passions and creativity make us unique and give us pleasure. What can you do in this situation to bring fun and joy into your life?

SUPPORT and STILLNESS

Step 4

Now is the time to reach out for support if the situation calls for it. Go to those whom you can trust and feel completely safe and supported by.

The final step towards maintaining balance in your life today is to take a moment of stillness and come into the present moment with renewed intentions and peace of mind. Balance will be waiting for you on the other side of this brief but very important meditative moment.

Build a supportive community where abundance can flourish
(root chakra)

Appreciate pleasure and joy in your life (sacral chakra)

Liberate personal power and energy to fuel ambition and
desires (solar plexus chakra)

Accept love with an open heart and live with compassion
and gratitude (heart chakra)

Nurture self-expression, speak your truth in order to live an
authentic experience (throat chakra)

Cultivate a vivid imagination, intuition and clarity through
observation (third-eye chakra)

Expand your awareness, find peace and observe oneness
(crown chakra)

....

Acknowledgements

This book is dedicated to my first child who made it earthside.
Adam, you made me a mumma and in doing so you set in motion
a chapter of life filled with some of the most contented, fulfilled
and joyful days I have ever experienced. Every day I spend with
you fills me with endless love and gratitude. You are truly loved.

In the early days of mothering you taught me the art of living a
balanced life, and for this I thank you and gift this book to you for
your onward journey through life. May your adventures be filled
with endless wonder, your heart be filled with gratitude and your
being know creativity and stillness, with intuition as your guide.
This is my wish for you.